Sports Cupping

A Beginner's Guide to Cupping Therapy for
Athletes at Any Level

Maggie Hansen

Table of Contents

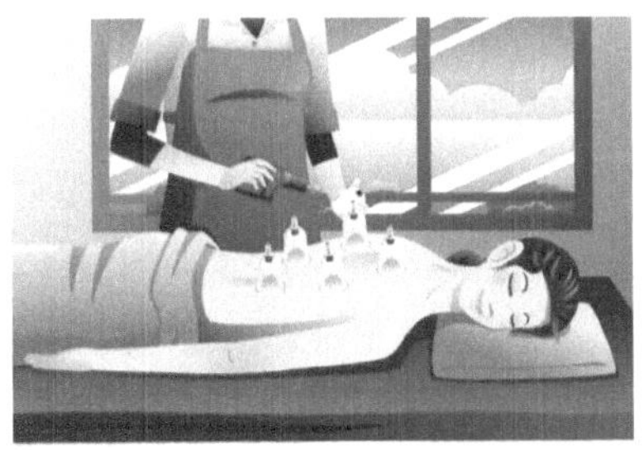

Introduction

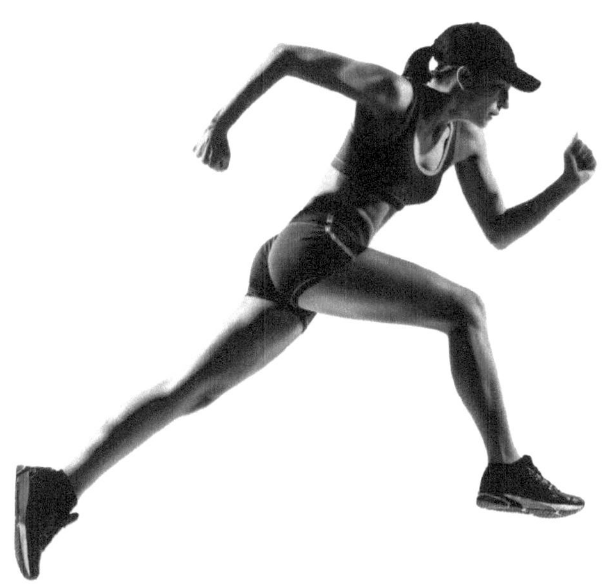

Athletes go through a lot. Through training and competitions, they push their minds and bodies to the limit, grit their teeth through the pain, rest, and then do it all over again. Active people who don't play their sport professionally are also often intense and have goals they want to meet. Getting hurt is just part of the game, but without proper treatment, a seemingly-minor injury can debilitate an athlete for good.

What's the best way to treat a sports-related injury? In Western medicine, RICE is upheld as the gold standard. That stands for rest, ice, compression, and elevation. While these treatments can be effective, they often only treat the symptom and not the real problem. However, in Traditional Chinese Medicine (TCM), no injury is surface-level. To really encourage healing and build strength, you have to get to the core of the condition.

In this book, you'll learn about the Traditional Chinese Medicine system and what it means to "treat the root." Every organ, bodily function, and tissue in the body is connected, and by stimulating certain points, a therapist can treat a myriad of problems and alleviate symptoms like soreness, pain, and numbness. Cupping, which is the use of special cups and suction on the pressure points, is an ancient treatment used in China and other countries. Athletes like Michael Phelps receive cupping, and studies have shown it might be effective on conditions as varied as nausea and anxiety.

What else can you expect from this book? You'll find a detailed explanation on the history of cupping, complementary treatments, and the supplies you'll need. There are also guides on how to cup specific injuries like sprains, cramps, fractures, and more. We'll also cover health conditions that can affect an athlete's performance, like insomnia, asthma, and anxiety. The information in this book is intended for educational purposes only and does not constitute actual medical advice. If you believe you might have an injury stemming from your athletic activity, you should go to a professional and get a diagnosis before attempting any treatments.

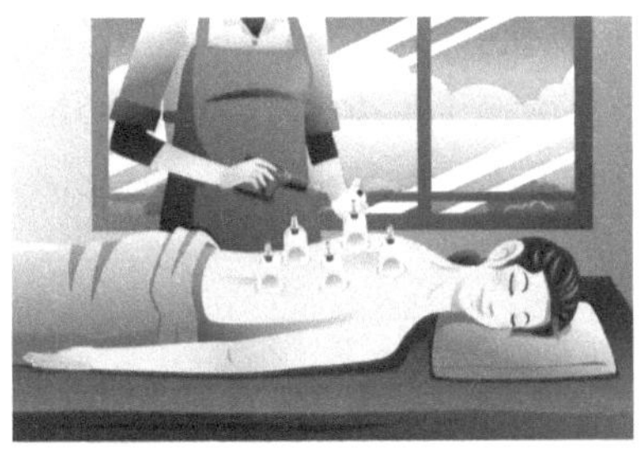

Chapter 1

Traditional Chinese Medicine 101

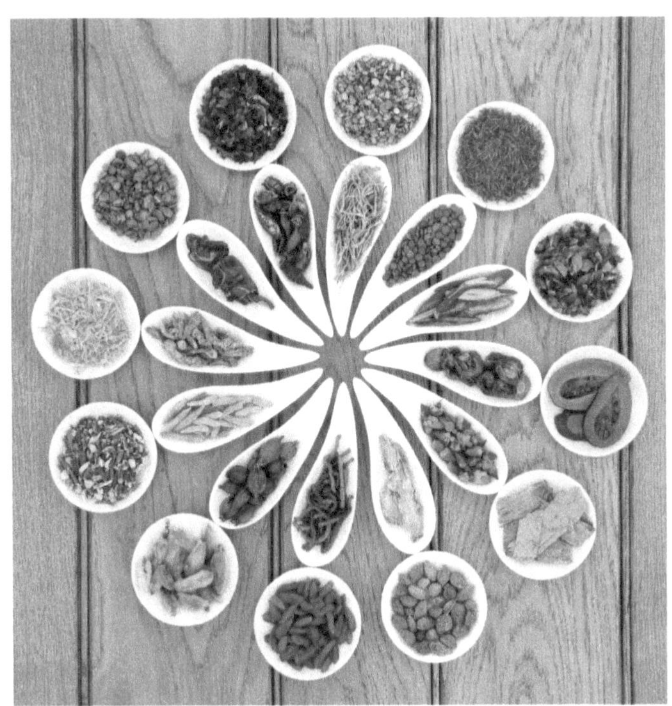

When it comes to history, we're often told that while we should learn from it, the best always lies in the future. That certainly seems true when we look at technology and the medical field, but even our modern hospitals with robots that can perform surgery often disappoint. That's when people turn to the ancient past for help.

Traditional Chinese medicine has been around for thousands of years, and research has shown that a lot of its teachings are actually accurate. While giving different names to conditions and parts of the anatomy, the foundation is based on careful observation and experimentation. Men like Shennong, a king who has since been promoted to a deity, supposedly ate hundreds of herbs to judge their medicinal value. Today, we don't have to do that, because we have thousands of years' worth of traditional healing to draw from.

While this book is about cupping, it's important to have some idea of Traditional Chinese Medicine's main principles. There are several terms that will come up again and again, so it's worth taking the time now to learn.

The concept of qi

"Qi" is the key term in Traditional Chinese Medicine. The word represents energy of all kinds, including flesh and blood. All of life is a collection of qi and when it's in a healthy balance within a person's body, that person is healthy.

The other aspect of qi you should know about is "yin and yang." These represent opposite manifestations of qi. Yin is solid, heavy, cold, moist, dark, and cooling. Yang is hollow, light, hot, dry, warming, and bright. They are in constant motion, adjusting to each other, and coming together in harmony. When they aren't in perfect balance within the body, it causes pain and illness.

Yin and yang can either be deficient or in excess. Yin, which manifests as positive things that the body and mind need, can be reduced and throw off the yin-yang balance. The yin of every organ (kidney, heart, spleen, etc.) can become deficient, and certain symptoms arise that let a therapist know where the source of the problem is. To treat yin deficiency, different herbs, cupping treatments, and diet can be applied to "tonify" or replenish yin.

Excessive yang reduces yin and the body's overall qi. Yang manifests as things like toxins, too much of an emotion, too much heat, and even too much sex. When balanced, yang isn't necessarily fundamentally bad, but when there's too much of it, it throws off the body's harmony.

The six evils

There are six evils that damage the yin-yang balance. They can be either external or internal. Athletes have an increased risk for injury because they're working their bodies harder than sedentary people, so even if they were perfectly healthy and resistant to the evils, overtraining or an accident could cause injury. We won't get into too much detail in this book, because these evils usually result in illness and aren't specific to sports injuries, but we'll provide a brief description:

Wind

Wind is the most "important" evil because in Traditional Chinese Medicine, it is believed to cause most diseases. It makes yang grow, throwing off yin. There are sub-winds that each bring their own unique problems, such as chills and an aversion to cold (wind-cold) or redness and fever (wind-heat). Wind tends to attack the lungs.

Cold

This evil damages yang and causes blood and qi stagnation. Like with wind, therapists look at the specific symptoms to determine where the "cold evil" is targeting its attack.

Damp

Damp also damages the yang and causes heaviness and stagnation. When dampness is internal, it can be a sign of a disease like chronic fatigue or something as serious as lymphoma.

Heat fire

This evil damages yin and tends to arise during the summer when the temperature is hot, but it can also originate deep within the body and organs. The skin is easily affected by heat and becomes red, itchy, and rashy.

Summer heat

An external evil that attacks yin, summer heat is different from heat because it *only* occurs during the summer. It is the only evil that does not have an internal counterpart. Symptoms of summer heat include fever, fatigue, dizziness, and so on.

Dryness

The dryness evil tends to attack during the fall system, and affects the lungs most strongly. It also manifests as dry skin, dry hair, dry eyes, and thirst.

The organs and emotions

In Traditional Chinese Medicine, each organ is associated with an emotion, so if there's something wrong with it, you'll feel an excess of a certain feeling. It works in the reverse, too: if you feel an excessive amount of a certain emotion, it can damage the corresponding organ. Understanding this connection can help everyone - including athletes - identify what might be troubling them:

The heart - *joy*
The kidneys - *fear*
The lungs - *sadness/grief*
The liver - *anger/frustration*
The spleen - *worry/overthinking*

The power of pressure points

The body's qi all flows through a series of pathways called "meridians" or "pressure points." These are like gates that can be opened (healthy) or blocked (unhealthy). Ideally, you want all of the gates opened, so qi can move freely through the body to support the organs and bodily functions. If those pathways are blocked, illness, pain, and other health problems result. You can remove those blockages by applying pressure to the pressure points.

Where do you find these points? They are found in natural indents (like between joints, in the temple, in the arch of the foot, etc.) all over the body. To treat an area, you apply pressure to the pressure points close by, but the points that are further away may be actually more powerful. Known as "distal points," these pressure points can open up whole channels of qi. The hand has lots of distal points that correspond to areas in the back, head, and feet, while the bottom of the foot is basically a microcosm of the organs.

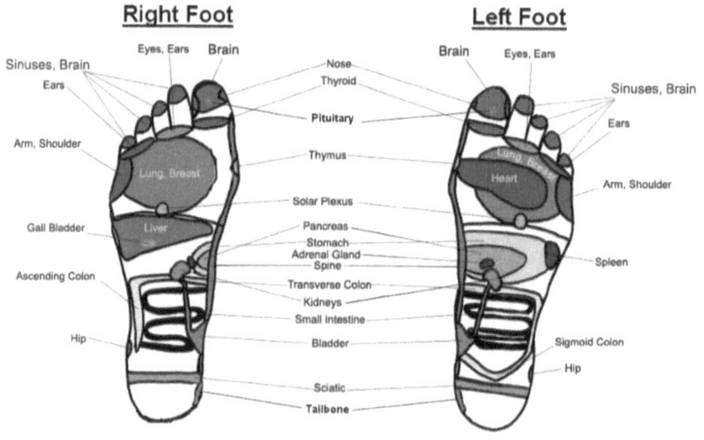

In Traditional Chinese Medicine, pressure points are all named and labeled. Today, the naming system consists of abbreviations for the area of the body that the point corresponds to and a number. For example, GB-21 means that point is the 21st point for the gallbladder meridian. The point is found in the shoulder because that meridian runs across the shoulders, top of the head, back of the neck, and forehead. This book will use the standard names, so you can look them up if you want more clarification about their location.

When you do further research, you might come across the term "ashi point." This isn't a specific point, but rather refers to the area where pain or discomfort is located. For example, if you're experiencing foot pain, the ashi point is the place that feels the most tender.

Point glossary

Lung - abbreviated as LU/there are 11 LU points in the body

Large Intestine - abbreviated as LI (in other sources, sometimes CO for "colon")/ there are 20 LI points in the body

Stomach - abbreviated as ST/ there are 45 ST points in the body

Spleen - abbreviated as SP/ there are 21 SP points in the body

Heart - abbreviated as HE (in other sources, sometimes as H or HT)/ there are 9 HE points in the body

Small Intestine - abbreviated as SI

Urinary Bladder - abbreviated as UB (in other sources, sometimes as BL for "bladder")

Gallbladder - abbreviated as GB

Kidney - abbreviated as KI (in other sources, sometimes as K)

Pericardium - abbreviated as PC (in other sources, sometimes as P)

Triple Burner - abbreviated as TB (in other sources, sometimes as TW for "triple-warmer" or SJ for San Jiao)

Liver - abbreviated as LV (in other sources, sometimes as LR)

Governing Vessel - abbreviated as GV (in other sources, sometimes as DU)

Conception - abbreviated as CV (in other sources, sometimes as REN)

Extra Points - abbreviated as Ex

Summary

It's challenging to summarize an entire system of medicine in just a few pages, but I think I've provided the gist of it. The body is sustained by "qi," which represents the energy in all living things. Without qi, life wouldn't exist. Qi has two parts - yin and yang - that balance each other out. Qi flows through the body in pathways, or meridians that can be accessed by stimulating certain points on the body. These are known as pressure points.

When yin and yang are unbalanced in your body, health problems arise. Six "evils" can cause this imbalance and make the body vulnerable to disease and injury, though external factors like a bad fall also cause injury. To speed up healing, therapists stimulate pressure points which are labeled according to their relevant organ. This stimulation provides a myriad of benefits and allows qi to flow freely again.

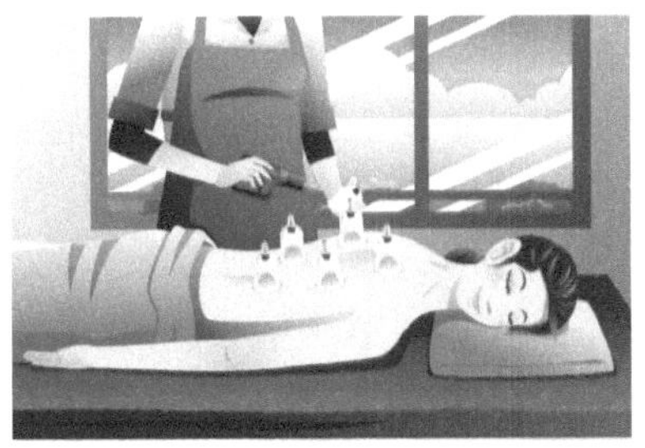

C h a p t e r   2

Cupping 101

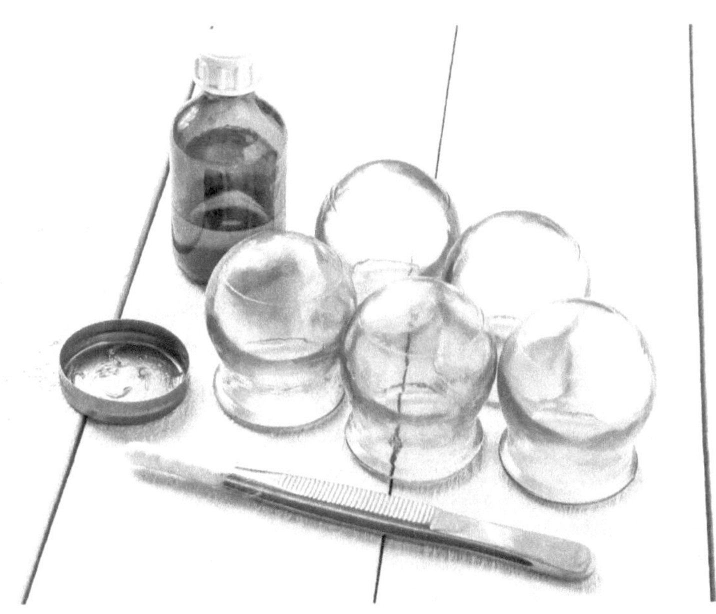

Cupping stimulates pressure points to heal the body and encourage proper organ function. It's different than massage, which pushes *in* to the body. The goal of cupping is to draw *outwards*. Through suction, healthy blood is drawn to the cupped pressure point, so it can flow through that meridian. Stagnant toxins are also pulled to the area, which encourages the body to get rid of them properly.

Athletes usually receive "dry cupping." The therapist gets out a set of clean and sterilized glass cups in different sizes. They light a cotton ball or a piece of paper and hold it with a pair of long tweezers, so they don't burn their fingers. This goes into the glass cup, where it heats up the glass. When the therapist decides it's at the right temperature, they remove the flame, blow it out, and then place the cup mouth-side down on the patient's body. The heat creates suction, which draws blood to the surface and pulls the skin up.

Cupping benefits

Why would a person receive cupping? Why would an athlete? There are a lot of reasons. Athletes experience a lot of pain from sore muscles and joints, and cupping can increase endorphins, the body's natural pain-reliever. Cupping can also reduce inflammation and joint stiffness. The suction pulls muscle and tissue up from the bones, allowing blood and oxygen-rich lymph to flow to the affected area. The healing process speeds up, while nutrients from the lymph strengthen the immune system and protect the athlete from infections.

During hard workouts, an athlete's body receives a build-up of uric acid, lactic acid, cholesterol, and calcium deposits. These inhibit tissue and muscle recovery following an injury. A cupping treatment breaks down these toxins, so it's easier for the body to flush them out. The body is now able to heal itself properly, while the athlete's muscles and tissue are stronger than ever.

The other benefit from cupping is treatment for myofascial pain syndrome. This is a disorder when pressure on certain muscle points results in pain from another body part, seemingly-unrelated. It occurs in athletes who overuse their muscles or repeat an injury. Cupping relieves pain, increases flexibility, and also treats muscle spasms after intense workouts. This appeals to athletes wanting to improve their performance.

Cupping can treat a variety of other health problems that afflict everyone and not just athletes. These conditions include:

- Colds and congestion
- Headaches
- Anxiety
- Insomnia
- Heartburn
- Stomach and digestion issues
- Arthritis

In this book, I'll provide guides on athlete-specific problems like leg cramping and foot pain, but there will also be walkthroughs on other problems athletes face that inhibit their performance or result from activity, like anxiety, insomnia, and nausea.

Types of cupping

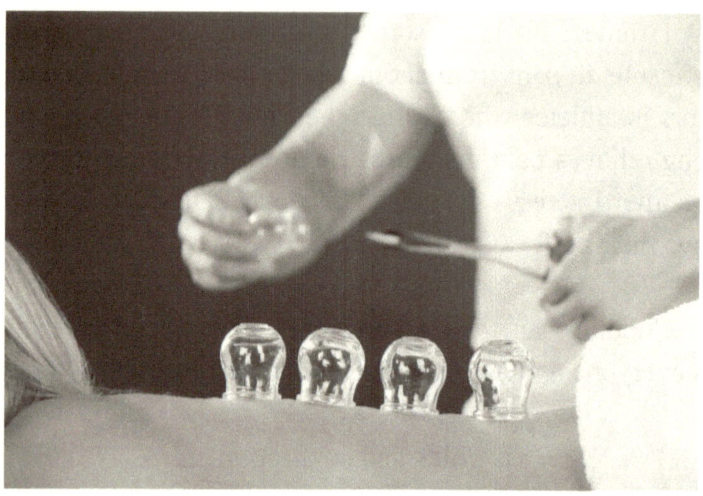

The most basic form of dry cupping consists of glass cups heated by flame. The cup remains stationary on the body for the length of time prescribed by the therapist. There are other forms of cupping, however, that athletes use frequently:

Vacuum cupping

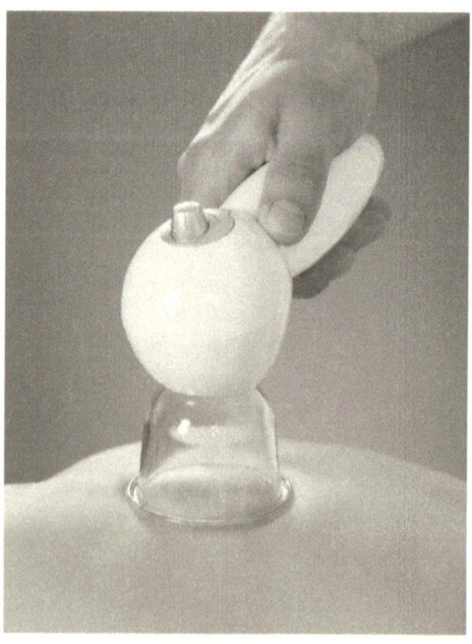

The main difference between vacuum cupping and traditional dry cupping is that vacuum cupping does not use flame. Instead, suction is created with a hand pump or suction bulbs on the cup itself. Therapists use plastic, rubber, or silicone cups instead of glass. Using the hand pump or bulbs gives the therapist total control over the amount of suction. It's considered safer than traditional dry cupping because it doesn't involve fire.

Massage cupping

The cups are moved on the body for this treatment. The therapist applies oil to the body first, so the cups glide smoothly. Massaging the body through cupping helps qi and blood circulate better through the body. Because glass is not a very flexible material, plastic, rubber, or silicone cups are often used instead.

Flash cupping

Flash cupping lasts only a few seconds and is usually done on the face, because this type of cupping doesn't leave marks. Suction is applied for just a few seconds several times during a session.

Herbal cupping

Herbs are boiled in water and then the cup, usually bamboo, sits in the water for 2-3 minutes. The cup is drained, and then the therapist covers the mouth with a wet towel to create steam. The cup is placed and held on the body for 30 seconds or so, until suction forms, and the cup sticks by itself.

Wet cupping

Wet cupping, also known as "hijama" in Arabic, involves normal cupping plus bleeding. It's a traditional Islamic practice. After cupping for 3 minutes, the therapist removes the cup and makes a small incision on the part of the body that was just cupped. Then, that area is covered with another cup. Stagnant blood and other toxins are pulled out of the incision, filling the cup. After 5-10 minutes, the therapist removes the cups and disposes of the blood. The incisions are cleaned and bandaged. To clean the cups, therapists must use a high-level disinfectant after removing the blood with hot water and soap. Athletes do receive hijama, though it isn't practiced very much in North America.

Needle cupping

Needle cupping combines dry cupping and acupuncture. The therapist performs acupuncture, leaving the needle in the skin. The heated cup is placed *over* the needle and maintained for a certain length of time.

Water cupping

The rarest form of cupping, a therapist fills a cup ⅓ of the way with warm water, then lights a piece of cotton or paper. They put the cotton into the water and then turn the cup over on the patient's body. Ideally, they move so quickly that no water spills out.

History

No one knows for sure which civilization invented cupping. It appeared in ancient China, Egypt, and the Middle East before spreading to Europe and the Americas. Before glass and plastic, therapists used bamboo and even the horns of animals. Cupping served the dual purpose of cleansing the body from physical and spiritual contaminants. Let's take a closer look at how cupping developed.

Ancient cupping

The earliest records of cupping in China go back 3,000 years, when it was used to treat pulmonary tuberculosis. Its most famous early advocate - alchemist and herbalist GeHong - wrote "A Handbook of Prescriptions for Emergencies," where he described using cupping to drain pus from blisters. The phrase, "Acupuncture and cupping, more than half of the ills cured," is attributed to him. Later, during the Tang dynasty, cupping treatment expanded into stomach pain, dizziness, and headaches. Neighboring countries like Korea, Japan, and Vietnam also practiced cupping, as archaeologists have discovered tools.

Hieroglyphic evidence shows that Egypt began cupping around the same time as China. The Ebers Papyrus, an ancient medical text, describes the use of the treatment. Hippocrates traveled to Egypt and learned cupping, which he practiced upon his return to Greece in 400 B.C.

In ancient Persia, wet cupping was known as "al hijama." Described in the Quran, al hijama is advocated by Muhammad as "the best of remedies." Islamic groups like the Arabs and Turks practiced wet cupping for both spiritual and physical reasons.

Cupping in the West

The Western world practiced cupping because of its use in Greece. Through the 1800's, it was a common treatment in Europe and the United States. To prove cupping's effectiveness, China collaborated with the Soviet Union on a massive study. The positive results inspired all Chinese hospitals to allow cupping as an official treatment option.

In Europe and North America, however, cupping fell out of style as new medications and technology appeared. Because of its association with spirituality, Western science turned its nose up at cupping. Relegated to the ranks of "alternative medicine," most people weren't familiar with it unless they sought it out. That changed once celebrities like Gwyneth Paltrow and Michael Phelps began appearing in magazines with the marks of cupping. In 2016, all kinds of athletes sported the tell-tale bruises, and the media began publishing more stories on cupping. One of their key questions: does it actually work?

Does science support cupping?

There aren't a lot of studies on cupping, so it's difficult to say definitely if it works or not. The studies that are out there, however, are promising. In 2015, a report appearing in the Journal of Traditional Chinese Medical Sciences showed that cupping might be linked to pain relief and acne reduction. Other studies have shown that dry cupping can reduce nausea and anxiety, and possibly the inflammation of muscles and joints. The latter result is especially interesting to athletes, who often suffer from inflamed muscles and joints.

Why is it hard to produce studies on cupping? It's because of the process modern science uses: the randomized-controlled trial. In this trial, participants are divided into groups where one receives the actual treatment and another receives a placebo. However, there is no placebo for cupping. It isn't something you can really "fake." Researchers use different methods to test cupping's effectiveness, but all the conclusions say something along the lines of, "More research is needed." Due to this lack of research, most medical doctors don't advocate cupping. Many see it as a pseudoscience and useless health trend promoted by celebrities.

Cupping risks

Another reason why doctors are wary of cupping is because of the risks it comes with. By its definition, wet cupping is riskier than dry cupping. This is because the therapist actually cuts into your skin. The risks of infection are significantly increased. That's why it's especially important to see a licensed professional who meets the highest hygiene standards if you're considering wet cupping.

Most dry-cupping accidents involve burns from the fire. The glass can be heated too much and leave painful blisters on the skin. Other common complaints from traditional dry cupping *and* vacuum cupping include inflammation, capillary rupture, blood clots, and soreness.

Cupping patients also risk aggravating their problem further if they don't have a well-educated therapist or if they fail to tell their therapist enough about their health status. You should not receive cupping if you are tired, hungry, or have a fever. If your skin is bruised, broken, or swollen, you shouldn't receive cupping in that area.

There are certain people who are advised against cupping altogether:

- Pregnant women
- People with skin allergies
- Those with a bleeding disease
- Those on a blood-thinning medication
- Under 4-years old
- Elderly and frail

The last risk that comes with cupping is the temptation to forgo other treatments. In cases of terminal illness, replacing another treatment with cupping could be fatal. That's why doctors are generally skeptical about cupping because of how it's upheld in the media and by celebrities as some kind of "cure-all." It isn't and should only be undertaken by those who are aware of its limitations, risks, and what other options are out there for their condition.

Summary

This chapter covered all the basics of cupping, which is a therapy with lots of benefits like reduced inflammation, better circulation of healing nutrients, pain relief, and more. It can treat virtually any kind of health problem like headaches, insomnia, anxiety, and sports-related injuries. There are several types of cupping, including the traditional dry cupping which uses a glass cup and flame to create suction on the skin. This type is dangerous without a professional. The most popular cupping these days is vacuum cupping, which uses silicone, plastic, or rubber cups. No fire is required, just suction from a pump or bulb. In this book, we'll refer to it as "cupping."

Cupping has existed for thousands of years and has been making a comeback in the West. The science on cupping's benefits and risks is shaky, mostly because it's very difficult to conduct studies on the therapy. Reported risks include blood clots and soreness (the cupping we use in this book is the least risky), and doctors are concerned that people might substitute other types of treatment with cupping. This is why it's so important to talk to a professional before undergoing this treatment.

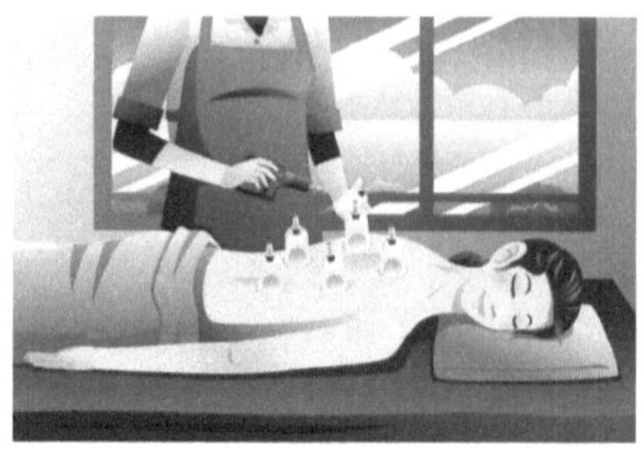

Chapter 3

Complementary Treatments

Cupping is rarely practiced by itself. There is almost always some other element of Traditional Chinese Medicine incorporated, like acupuncture or regular massage. The idea is that while one treatment is effective, adding even more can only increase qi and the body's ability to heal. It's important that the treatments don't counteract each other, so therapists are educated on what works best together. There are nine treatments that are either used in conjunction with cupping or are similar to cupping.

Acupuncture

Acupuncture is arguably the oldest physical therapy in the world. China has used it for 8,000 years. By inserting very thin needles into the skin, therapists stimulate pressure points all over the body to relieve pain and treat every type of disease. Acupuncture has been studied more than cupping, and research suggests that the treatment is effective. Whether or not that effect is purely placebic is impossible to know. Acupuncture is frequently performed after dry cupping, and you'd be hard-pressed to find a cupping therapist who didn't also offer acupuncture.

Acupressure

Acupressure is essentially the same as cupping and acupuncture, but instead of needles or cups, therapists use their hands and elbows. Using simple pressure, blocked meridians are opened and a person's qi flows freely again. It's very safe and people frequently use it on themselves to relieve nausea, heartburn, etc., since those points are found on body parts they can access easily.

Electroacupuncture

Electroacupuncture begins like normal acupuncture, with needles inserted into the body. A device that produces continuous electrical pulses gets clipped to a pair of needles, so the current passes between one needle to the other. The current stimulates a wide area of the meridian. This electricity works the pressure points continuously, boosting the treatment's effectiveness. It's also said to encourage a higher endorphin production that stays in the bloodstream longer. This results in better pain relief. For those afraid of needles, electroacupuncture can also be performed with electrode pads. This method is known as "transcutaneous electrical nerve stimulation."

Dry needling

Though it sounds like it would be similar to acupuncture and it does make use of a thin needle that's inserted into the skin, they are two different treatments. Dry needling was developed much more recently and is used to improve theneuro-musculo-skeletal function. When an athlete is injured, the damaged tissue becomes inflamed. The tissue proceeds to protect itself and begins to produce scar tissue. This prevents the muscles and tissue from working as well as they should. Dry needling seeks to penetrate affected muscles and tissue, which are known as "trigger points." The needle insertion restores normal function and movement to the area, though many say it's very painful at first. Dry needling is rarely performed by itself and is part of a longer course of treatment for injured athletes.

Aromatherapy

Although there's no translation of "aromatherapy" in Traditional Chinese Medicine, it's definitely a part of ancient healing traditions. The definition of aromatherapy is the utilization of extracted essences from aromatic plants to promote good health. These "essences" are more commonly-known as essential oils and have the power to encourage relaxation, improve breathing, and more. Therapists will often rub essential oil blends into a patient's skin, and they breathe in the fragrance that way. Diffusers are also popular. Diffusers are appliances specifically designed to turn water and drops of essential oil into fragrant mist, and you'll see them a lot at massage therapists' offices.

Chinese herbal medicine

The Chinese have used the healing power of herbs for centuries, while research using modern scientific methods has proved the effectiveness of the system. Herb blends are used in both modern and traditional treatments, and every cupping and acupuncture therapist will have some education in herbal medicine. Herbs are offered in raw form or as supplements. They can also be used as poultices (mashed-up herbs rubbed directly on the skin) or in plasters. You'll also frequently see herbs used in place of ice. While in Western sports medicine, ice is used to reduce inflammation and swelling, Traditional Chinese Medicine uses the consumption of herbs. Ice is too cold and stagnates the blood, while herbs tackle the problem internally.

A typical treatment lasts 1 month to 1 year, while the type of herb you use depends on your condition. The most effective way to use herbal medicine is to take blends of several herbs, since they work best together. Here's a list of the ten most important herbs to know:

> ***Ginseng*** - Used as an aphrodisiac and treatment for PMS, high blood pressure, low energy, and brain power.

> ***Dang Gui (Angelica Sinesis)*** - Used to treat high blood pressure, infertility, and stiff muscles.

> ***Reishi mushrooms*** - Used to strengthen the immune system, for female sexual dysfunction, and to improve insomnia.

Cordyceps mushrooms - Used to improve immune system, enhance athletic stamina, and improve liver function.

Peach seed - Improves blood circulation and digestive functions.

Ma Huang (Ephedra Sinica) - One of the oldest chinese herbs, it treats congestion, asthma, and other lung problems.

Bupleurum - Treats liver diseases, ulcers, and mental disorders.

Safflower - Treats stagnation, swelling, and stomach pain.

White peony root - Treats lower-body cramping and muscle spasms.

Licorice root - Removes toxins and treats heartburn, the flu, the common cold, and depression.

Astragalus - Strengthens the immune system, improves digestion, and prevents infections.

Ginkgo biloba - Treats heart and lung problems, and improves cognitive function.

Lotus seed - Improves kidney and spleen function.

Ciwujia (Siberian ginseng) - Regulates nervous, endocrine, and cardiovascular system.

How to choose the best brands

Finding good herbal formulations can be tricky. When you're researching online, be sure to only trust websites run by health associations, health professionals, and universities. It's also a good idea to do your research on free non-profit or government-run sites instead of ones with lots of advertisements. If the site needs to generate ad revenue, odds are they're going to be a little biased about some of the supplements they're selling.

When you find a formulation, be wary of buzzwords like "natural." These words don't really mean anything. It's a really good idea to look for brands that follow Good Manufacturing Practices regulations, which is enforced by the FDA and helps monitor the quality of herb and vitamin supplements. It looks at factors like contamination, since the amount of contamination in these products made the news a few years back. One gingko product ended up being contaminated with black walnut, which can cause skin reactions and respiratory distress. To find better brands, look for markers that show the supplement has been tested by an independent organization, like NSF International or Natural Products Association.

Before taking any herbs, talk to your doctor to make sure you're educated on side effects and possible interactions with other medications you're on.

Where can you get Chinese herbs?

Acupuncturists and practitioners of Chinese medicine will most likely have a pharmacy you can buy from. If they are too expensive, you can buy online, but again, you want to be very careful. Here are some online resources that appear legitimate:

Spring Winds Herbs

Their website states they have the most rigorous pesticide testing program "in the industry." They also pay close attention to the species of herbs so they can correctly label every product. Their Canadian distributor is called Organic Chinese Herbs.

Dr. Shen

Made in the US, Dr. Shen products use whole herbs, which are submitted for lab testing. Their partners are all GMP-compliant and the final batch is tested for things like heavy metals, mold, and other contaminants. They don't use any dyes, chemical solvents, or sugar coatings. All their herbal supplements are gluten-free.

Pacific Herbs

This company states that they use the herbs approved by the Australian government and the Japanese governmental agencies which have the most rigid standards in the world.

Moxibustion

This treatment essentially combines acupuncture with herbal medicine. It's intended to enhance the effectiveness of acupuncture and cupping. The therapist rolls herbs into a ball (this is called the "moxa") and sticks it on top of the inserted acupuncture needle. They light the moxa on fire. This sends detoxifying heat and energy down through the needle into the pressure point. It strengthens the blood that's been brought to the area by cupping or acupuncture. With indirect moxibustion, the therapist puts the moxa on a stick, lit it, and holds it close to the area, but doesn't actually use it on an inserted needle. Moxibustion is used frequently for patients with swollen joints and fatigue.

Studies have shown that acupuncture combined with moxibustion is effective at treating athletes with ankle ligament injury. Another study specifically about cupping and moxibustion showed that after intense training, athletes treated with moxibustion and cupping experienced less fatigue than those who took a half-hour rest.

Kinesiology tape

Developed by chiropractors and acupuncturists in Japan, kinesiology tape is meant to encourage the body's natural ability to heal while extending the benefits of other treatments. Sumo wrestlers used it first and it came to international attention when Kerri Walsh won gold in the 2008 Olympics while sporting the tape on her shoulder while recovering from rotator-cuff surgery. The ultra-flexible, breathable tape can be cut in all sorts of shapes and sizes and used to reduce swelling, manage pain, and improve the performances of healthy, uninjured athletes.

The stretchy tape lifts the athlete's skin away from the muscle and the deeper tissues. This "lifting" effect is most apparent when swollen or bruised areas are taped. The inflammation and bruising is reduced, while the act of decompressing the tissue also reduces pain. Athletes also use tape to increase the brain's awareness of certain joints and muscles. By applying tape, the brain focuses on those areas because it senses touch. In theory, this enhances an athlete's control over their muscles and movements.

Gua sha

Translated into "rubbing congestion," gua sha is often known as "scraping" or "spooning" by Westerners. Using a tool with a smooth, blunt edge, gua sha therapists rub a patient's oiled skin to encourage healthy blood flow and remove toxins. Like cupping, it's supposed to encourage healing. The scraping leaves long, red scrape marks because the blood rises to just below the skin's surface, coloring it. Gua sha is used to treat tight muscles, pain, and stiffness. Other Asian countries have variations of the treatment. Vietnam calls it "ciao gio" and uses the edge of a coin.

Instrument Assisted Soft Tissue Mobilization (IASTM)

Based on gua sha, this treatment is intended for patients with soft tissue dysfunction and musculoskeletal conditions. Soft tissue is injured when an athlete gets a sprain, strain, ruptured blood vessel, bruise, or when a body part gets overused. Pain, bruising, swelling, and an inability to perform follow this injury. Through the body's natural healing process, scar tissues and adhesions form. The problem is that adhesions limit the athlete's movement in the affected area and can cause pain. Using tools made from stainless steel, plastic, or other materials, a therapist applies "microtrauma" to the affected area. This breaks up the adhesions (which can include scar tissue) and encourages healthy blood flow and muscle relaxation.

Neurokinetic therapy (NKT)

Developed in the 1980's, NKT is similar to massage therapy in that it seeks to correct movements that result in bad form, joint pain, and muscular pain. It consists of a series of muscle tests that reveal the incorrect movements, and then rehab exercises designed to retrain the brain on the correct ones. The MCC or motor control center of the brain (found in the cerebellum) is the part therapists focus on, since it's responsible for all the body's movements. You'll find NKT used in physical therapy and rehab situations. Runners and those with carpal tunnel syndrome often receive NKT, though any athlete can benefit from it. NKT can even be used to *prevent* sports injuries because it teaches the athlete the proper movements before the bad ones result in pain.

Summary

In this chapter, you learned about therapies similar to dry cupping or performed in place of it. Acupuncture is more ancient than cupping and is the most common therapy performed alongside cupping. Aromatherapy is also frequently used, as is herbal medicine. Moxibustion combines acupuncture and herbal medicine, as the therapist inserts a needle topped with a ball of herbs, which is lit on fire. Athletes might also use special kinesiology tape to help increase their flexibility. Gua sha and IASTM seem very similar as they both involve massage with a blunt instrument, but IASTM is specifically for soft tissue dysfunction and musculoskeletal conditions. The last treatment we discussed, neurokinetic therapy, is most commonly-used during rehab and physical therapy.

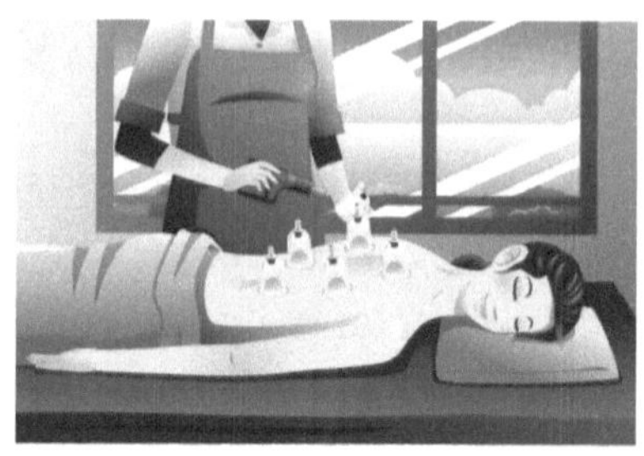

C h a p t e r   4

Cupping Supplies

Every good therapist needs good tools. When cupping, the cups are obviously the most important item, but they may be different depending on the type of cupping and the patient's needs. In this chapter, you'll learn about wet cupping supplies like the Plum Blossom needle, as well as how to choose the best cupping sets. All cupping sets leave marks - that's just the nature of the treatment - so you'll read about how the colors can vary and what they mean for your health. Therapists also need to think about massage oils and essential oils, which can enhance a patient's experience and boost cupping's effectiveness.

Wet cupping supplies

Therapists that practice wet cupping use cupping sets that are high-quality and can be cleaned and sterilized easily, because they collect blood during the treatment. Most materials are acceptable except bamboo. You'll see therapists using glass, plastic, and silicone mostly. We'll get into specific sets in the next section.

To make the small incisions, Plum Blossom needles are popular. They look a little like hammers, but instead of a round head, they have tiny spikes on them. The therapists "taps" on the skin to make the cuts. Look below to see an example of a Plum Blossom needle with seven "stars" or needles. You'll also find therapists using razor blades or surgical lancets.

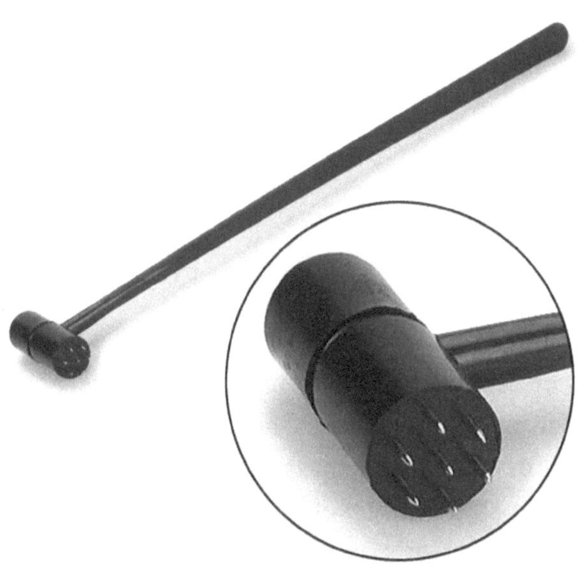

For cleaning, therapists who perform wet cupping need hot water, soap, and a high-level disinfectant. Disinfectants are graded according to the materials they come in contact with. Because wet cupping draws blood and/or pus, a high-level disinfectant is required. Ingredients will include hydrogen peroxide and glutaraldehyde.

Dry cupping supplies

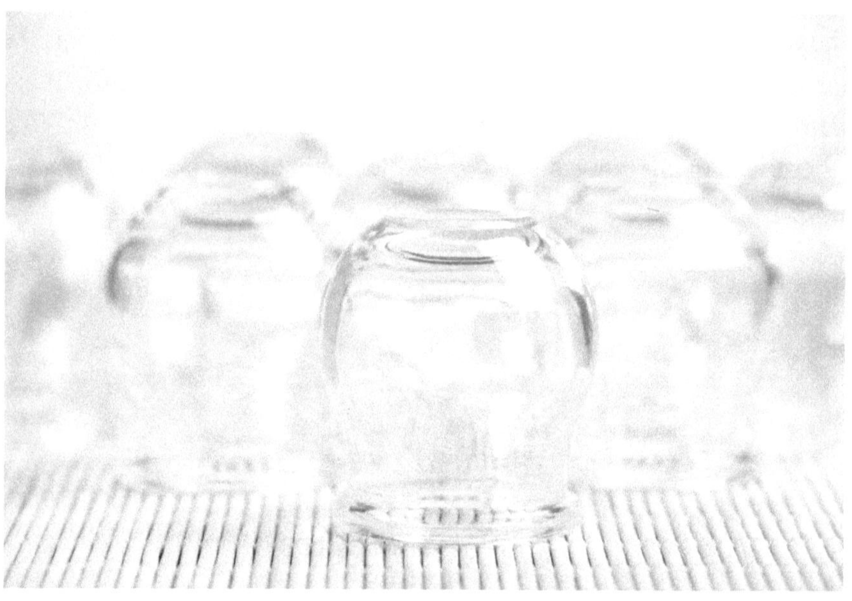

As you know, therapists have the choice between glass, plastic, rubber, or silicone cups. Glass is the only one you can use for traditional dry-cupping with flame. The benefit of glass is that it adheres to the skin really well, but on the other hand, you can't adjust the suction once it's on the patient's body. The heat - not the therapist - controls the vacuum. Another disadvantage is that glass breaks, while the other materials don't. Plastic is a popular material these days, and these sets let you control the suction with a hand pump. Sets include cups in a variety of sizes.

Rubber is another popular material and adjusting the suction is even easier than with plastic. The cups have little bulbs on top that you squeeze to create or release suction. They're very flexible and make massage cupping a breeze. Silicone cups have the same advantage, and they're also food-grade and easy to sterilize.

In China, you'll often see bamboo cups. However, they can't be sterilized properly, so they aren't safe. You also can't see how the skin is reacting to cupping because the cups aren't translucent.

What to look for in a cupping set

The two features you want to bear in mind when looking for a cupping set are size and suction control. Sets usually contain a few different sizes, and the more sizes you have, the more places on the body you can cup. Large cups are best on muscular, relatively-flat areas of the body like the back, stomach, chest, buttocks, and thighs. Medium-sized cups are used on the neck, arms, legs, and shoulders. For facial cupping and cupping between joints and bones, very small cups are ideal.

For suction, you want to have a lot of control. This lets you adjust based on what the patient is feeling and what suction strength is best for the condition you're treating. With glass sets, you don't have much control. More experienced therapists know how warm the glass should be, but once they apply the glass to the skin, their part ends. Cups that use hand pumps offer a lot of control and you can be very precise. Using cups that just have the bulb on top are also easy to adjust.

It's a small detail, but when you're shopping for cups, you should also take note of the cup's mouth. Narrow ones tend to be more effective, though they also cause a bit more discomfort and shouldn't be used for cupping on boils. You also want the edge of the mouth, the part that goes right against the skin, to be smooth. This decreases the amount of discomfort the patient feels, especially during massage cupping when the cup is sliding around.

Cupping set ideas

What cupping sets are the best-reviewed? We've compiled a list from buying guides on the web to let you know what's available:

Lure

Popular among therapists, professionals, and athletes, these silicone cups offer a lot of control over suction and movement. They are reasonably affordable, too, for the quality. Lure has a handful of sets like Edge, Bliss, and Zen. Edge has 6 cups (there is a 4-cup version, too) and is marketed as "Advanced Body Cupping." Bliss has 7 cups, which are designed for Face & Body. Zen is labeled as a 6-cup "Performance Body System." There's also a "Glam" set, which appears to be for facial cupping, and an "Energy" set. It isn't clear what that set does specifically, but they do appear to be just for stationary cupping and not massage.

Hansol Professional 17-piece

This brand makes the most popular set on Amazon. The cups are made of high-quality plastic in different sizes and come with a hand pump. The 17-piece set is around $30. Hansol also make a larger 30-piece set that includes magnetic inserts that enhance cupping's pain-relieving effectiveness. That costs $65.

Classic 4 Professional Medical

With just four cups, this is a really simple set that's great for beginners. It uses silicone and the sizes are small enough for your face. When you buy the set, you get video instructions on how to use the cups. At only $13, they're a steal. The manufacturer (Cupping Warehouse) also makes a Supreme 8 set, with eight cups instead of four so you can cup on larger areas of your body.

Endiglow Silicone

Another kit that's good for beginners, these cups are made with very soft edges, so you don't experience as much discomfort. Bear in mind that the weaker suction means less benefits, too.

Acu Supply 12-Piece

These high-quality glass cups are made with thick glass and textured finger grips for safety. Because these use fire, you can't apply them to yourself.

Do cups cause bruising?

Cupping leaves distinctive circular dark marks on the body. You've no doubt seen these on the backs, arms, and chests of Olympic athletes. They are called "bruises," but they're not actually true bruises. Normal bruises are caused by a trauma, like a bad fall, and the capillaries in the skin break. The marks caused by cupping are due to blood flow rushing to the area thanks to the suction.

What the different colors mean

Therapists can tell how healthy you are based on the color of your marks. Bright red means you're healthy and your blood doesn't have much stagnation. If the marks look scattered, the therapist will know there might be an issue with the organ closest to the marks' location. Moderately-dark marks indicate moderate stagnant, while very dark, practically-purple marks mean you have a lot of stagnation. If your skin is dark, all the marks are slightly darker and for those with olive skin, there might be a yellow or greenish tint. Below, you can see an example of cupping marks from an article by Dr. Jun Negoro:

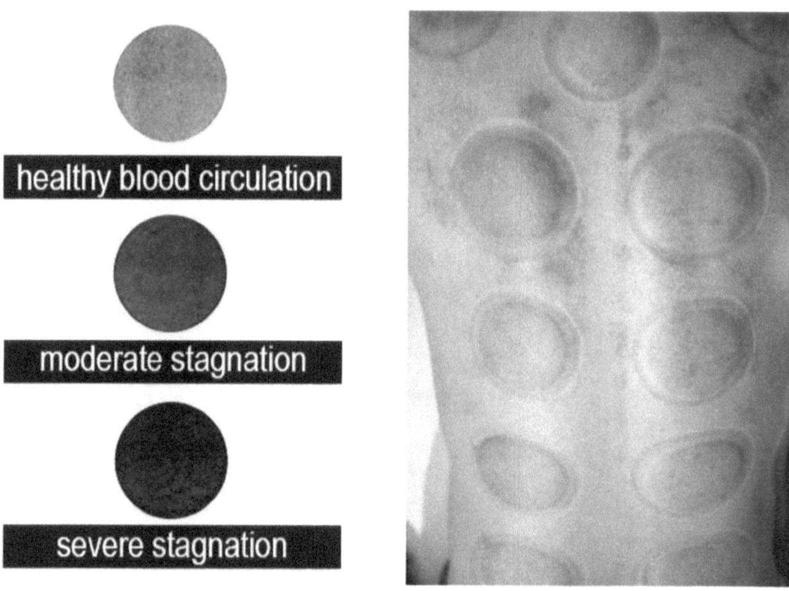

This patient has mostly bright red marks, which means they have healthy blood circulation. Athletes that compete in sports where they sweat a lot are likely to have paler marks, since toxins are flushed out in the sweat. Swimmers tend to have more pronounced marking, because of their exposure to pool chemicals.

There are other skin reactions therapists encounter that cause concern. Purple marks with black indicates very stagnant blood, while purple marks with plaque (scaly white marks) could mean the patient has an autoimmune illness. If the marks are light purple and blue with white plaque, they might have a kidney deficiency. For marks that are darker with white marks (purpura), you should see a doctor as soon as possible since it could be a result of a serious health problem.

The last two possible reactions are the most dramatic appearance-wise. If the patient has blisters within the cupping area, it means they have very dry skin. Their bodies don't have enough fluid, so they should hydrate right away. The therapist can continue cupping to improve the movement of bodily fluids. If the blisters are especially large or plentiful, the therapist might drain and bandage them. If nothing happens when you receive cupping - you just see a white mark - something is seriously wrong. It indicates a severe deficiency of qi and blood movement.

How long do marks last?

Cupping marks tend to fade in a few weeks, depending on how dark they are. The darker they are, the longer they take. Once the bruises fade, the therapist can cup on those areas again. As you continue your cupping treatment, the marks become progressively lighter.

To speed up the lightening process, patients have tried some simple techniques, such as "combing." First, they rub their marks with pure cabbage juice or an anti-bruising cream, which encourages circulation. Then they "comb" their marks (with an actual hair comb that's been sanitized) for 2 minutes. After a rest period of 2 minutes, they continue to comb for another 2 minutes. If the marks are sore, combing isn't the best option. Massaging the marks with the pads of your fingers will cause less discomfort. You should also be sure to drink lots of water right after a cupping treatment and throughout the next week, as hydration lightens the marks. Adding more iron-rich foods like spinach, grass-fed beef, pumpkin seeds, and eggs can help as well.

Cupping oils

Even if therapists aren't going to use massage cupping, they will apply oil to their patients. Cups adhere better to oiled skin. There are a lot of oils, so which is best? Most therapists use a blend of essential oils and a "carrier" oil. These are neutral oils that dilute the essential oil to a safe degree. Here's a list of the most common ones:

Coconut oil - Used in massage for centuries/Increases blood circulation and softens skin

Sweet almond oil - The mildest oil/Relieves inflammation and itchiness

Sesame oil - Used for Ayurvedic massage/Heals muscles and increases joint flexibility

Jojoba oil - Technically a wax/Doesn't feel greasy/Good for those with back acne

Apricot kernel oil - Similar to almond oil, good alternative for those with nut allergies/Doesn't feel greasy

No matter what carrier oil you use, you typically use 1 teaspoon of oil per 1 drop of essential oil.

Essential oils

Essential oils can play an important role in a cupping treatment. There are specific ones therapists will use to achieve different goals, and certain oils are especially good for athletes:

Peppermint

Peppermint essential oil can improve mental alertness and concentration, as well as relieve muscle pains. Its distinct Christmas-y scent can also reduce nausea and improve breathing.

Clove

Research on clove essential oil shows it can increase white blood cells and strengthen the immune system. It can also reduce inflammation and improve an athlete's flexibility.

Lemon

A "cheerful" oil, lemon is known to increase positive feelings while stimulating the nervous system. It can also be used to detoxify the body and prevent athlete's foot.

Eucalyptus

An oil with a strong scent, it can improve respiratory function as well as muscle inflammation and stiffness.

Lavender

The perfect oil for winding down, lavender can help steady nerves the night before a big competition, so the athlete gets the best sleep possible.

Best essential oil brands

When selecting an essential oil, there are a few things to look out for. The first is cost. If it's cheap, it probably isn't good.

Look at the highest-quality, most expensive oils and work your way down from there to figure out "how cheap is cheap." Essential oils should also not all be sold at the same price, because some are more rare than others. You should also check out the purity of the oil, with 100% being the gold standard. However, just because an oil is 100% pure doesn't mean it's the best. Look at the whole picture, like how they test the product. The best oils will go through the gas chromatography *and* mass spectrometry tests. These tests are abbreviated as GC/MS. The last criteria: buy organic.

Here are some recommended brands:

- Radha Beauty
- Plant Therapy
- Young Living
- Edens Garden

Summary

We covered a lot of information in this chapter, specifically what you need to perform cupping. When you're looking for a cupping set, size and suction control are the most important features. A good set will have a variety of sizes and give you maximum control. A soft edge is also a good idea. Besides your actual cups, you'll need massage oil and essential oils. Coconut oil is a classic and probably the most readily-available. An essential oil can add a lot to your cupping experience, so consider using one that promotes relaxation or helps your specific health issue.

The other topic we discussed in this chapter is the "bruises" that cupping leaves. These are actually not bruises, which are caused by trauma, but by the blood that flows to the cupped area because of the cup's suction. Therapists can learn how bad your blood stagnation is based on the color of the mark. If it's bright red, you're pretty healthy, but dark colors indicate that you will need more treatments. Bruises typically fade within a few weeks. You shouldn't cup on those areas until the marks have faded.

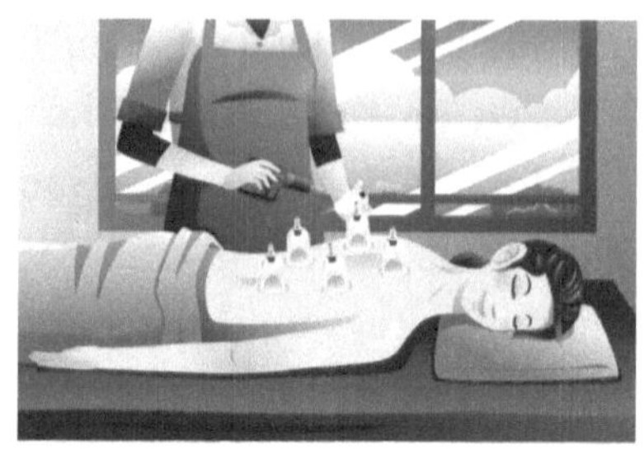

Chapter 5

Cupping the Most Common Injuries

No matter what sport an athlete engages in - soccer, football, rugby, basketball, tennis, or hockey - injuries are part of the game. A bad fall, overtraining, or just daily wear-and-tear can lead to sprains, strains, and more. In this chapter, you'll learn what the six most common sports injuries are and how cupping can help. The guides are for educational purposes only and do not replace actual medical advice. If you're in pain, you should consult your doctor first before attempting any treatment on your own.

The most common sports injuries

The following is a list of injuries athletes and active people are likely to experience at some point:

- Ankle sprain
- Groin pull
- Hamstring strain
- Shin splints

- Knee injury
- Tennis elbow

As you can see, most of these injuries are strains or pulls. When you stretch a ligament past its limit, it "sprains," or even becomes torn. Strains are injuries to muscle fibers or tendons. These are responsible for holding muscle to bone. Overstretching or overusing a muscle damages the fiber and/or tendon.

Who gets these injuries?

Ankle sprain - Pretty much any athlete can get an ankle sprain, because most sports involve foot work. Ankle sprains occur when you turn your foot inward, stretching the ligaments on the outside of your ankle, which aren't very strong.

Groin pull - Athletes that push off their legs side-to-side tend to get groin pulls. This includes baseball, hockey, basketball, and football players.

Hamstring strain - Three muscles make up the hamstring at the back of the thigh. Track running and sports with sprinting (soccer, basketball, football) cause hamstring strains.

Shin splints - Any athlete who runs can get shin splints, so you'll see it a lot in soccer players, tennis players, and basketball players. Dancers can get shin splints, too.

Knee injury - There are a few knee injuries an athlete can get. The ACL (anterior cruciate ligament) keeps the leg bone to the knee, and making a sudden stop, turn, or getting hit from the side can cause it to strain or even tear. A torn ACL requires surgery. When your kneecap and thigh bone engage in repetitive movements, it can damage the tissue underneath. Basketball, running, and volleyball can cause this injury, which is known as Patellofemoral syndrome.

Tennis elbow - Known as epicondylitis, tennis elbow is a tendon injury brought on by any repetitive movement of the arm, and not just tennis. Racquetball, squash players, and golfers get it, too. The pain tends to be on the outside of the arm, where the elbow and forearm meet.

Ankle sprain

The ankle is a relatively delicate part of the body - just one twist and you can seriously injure it. This is because the ligaments on the outer part of the ankle are relatively weak compared to the ligaments around it. If you feel pain and tenderness on the ankle, or see swelling and bruising, you have a sprain. If you felt or heard an audible pop when you turned your ankle, it's definitely sprained.

What points should you target?

GB-40 is a great place to apply light or medium cupping. If it's too painful to cup on the injured foot, cup on the other one. You can also use your finger on GB-40 and apply pressure until you feel a pulse. This is a good way to warm up the area and prepare it for cupping at a later time.

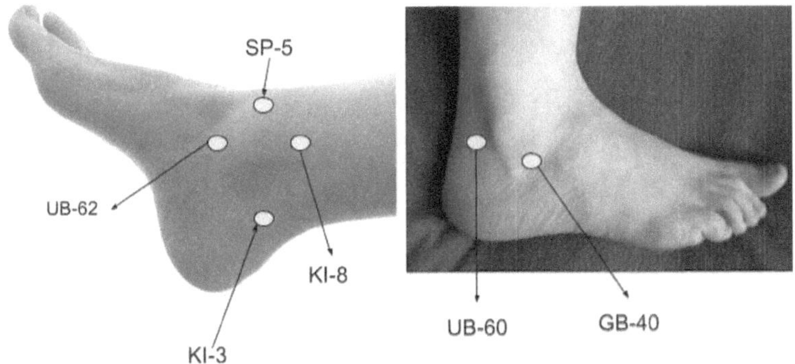

You can perform medium to strong cupping on SP-5, UB-60, UB-62, KI-8, and KI-3. These are all points in the foot, so if you feel too much discomfort, use light cupping for a shorter period of time.

Other treatments for ankle sprains

Traditional Chinese Medicine has a lot of herbal remedies for sprains. A therapist might recommend rubbing the ankle with a formulation of frankincense, myrrh, and safflower. This increases circulation to the area. A poultice of Three Yellow Powder, a famous blend, has a cooling effect on the swelling and the body. It is used instead of ice, because in Traditional Chinese Medicine, ice is too cold and stagnates the blood. You should also keep your weight off the ankle and engage in movement exercises, but not so it hurts. This prevents blood stagnation.

Groin pull

If you engage in a sport with a lot of running and jumping, you are at risk for overstretching or even tearing your groin or thigh muscles. Soccer and football players get them a lot, while they make up 10% of all hockey player injuries. Groin pulls make the area feel tender and painful. When you raise your knee or bring your legs together, you'll feel it. If you pull the muscle just a little, you'll experience some pain and loss of movement. If it's stretched further, the pain will be at a moderate level, and there might be tissue damage. If you heard or felt a pop or snap, you probably tore the muscle completely. That's the most severe type of groin injury.

What points should you target?

UB-28 and GB-28 are both points a therapist will cup. They are on the front and back, so the cupping treats both sides of the strain. Because these are sensitive areas, the therapist will probably warm the areas first by massaging with their hands.

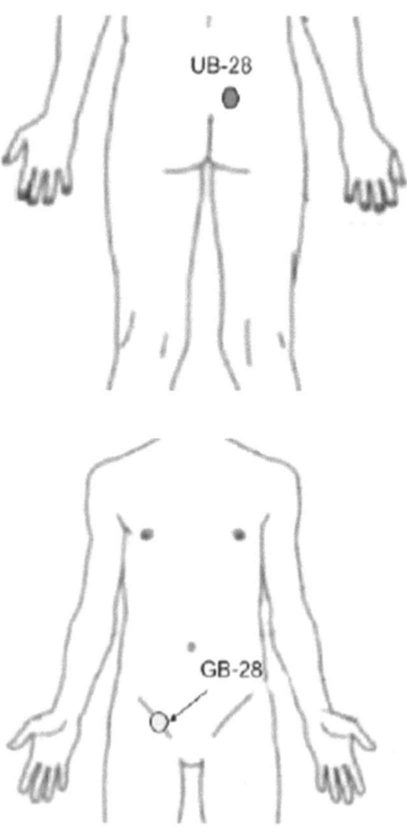

Other treatments for groin pulls

When you pull your groin muscle, it's important not to aggravate it any further. Playing through the pain can cause a Grade 1 pull to tear and become Grade 3. To reduce swelling, take a Three Yellow Powder formulation. Food with anti-inflammatories are helpful, as are any herbs that provide pain relief, such as corydalis root, turmeric, angelica, and safflower. To keep the blood circulating, engage in very careful stretches designed for those with groin injuries.

Hamstring strain

Your hamstring is made up of three muscles at the back of the knee. It allows you to extend your leg straight back and bend your knee. Athletes that use fast movements, like sprinters, frequently injure their hamstring muscles. Sometimes it's a minor pull that doesn't affect your walking, while at its worst, the tendon actually tears from the bone. Hamstring strains also occur from plain ol' fatigue: the quadriceps, which are the muscles at the front of the thigh, are stronger and let you work out longer. The hamstrings aren't as strong and get tired.

You will feel pain at the back of your thigh, from where the muscles link to the pelvis and knee. Spasms and stiffness are common, too, and walking will be difficult. You may also experience bruising and swelling in the area.

What points should you target?

Depending on how painful the hamstrings are, it's a good idea to cup on distal points. UB-65, UB-67, SI-1, LU-6, and KI-4 are all good points. These have an effect on the "tendinomuscular channel" (which just means it affects the tendons and muscles) and pain. You can also apply massage cupping on UB-36 through UB-40 on your hamstring, where the actual strain is found. Use light cupping at first and gauge how it feels.

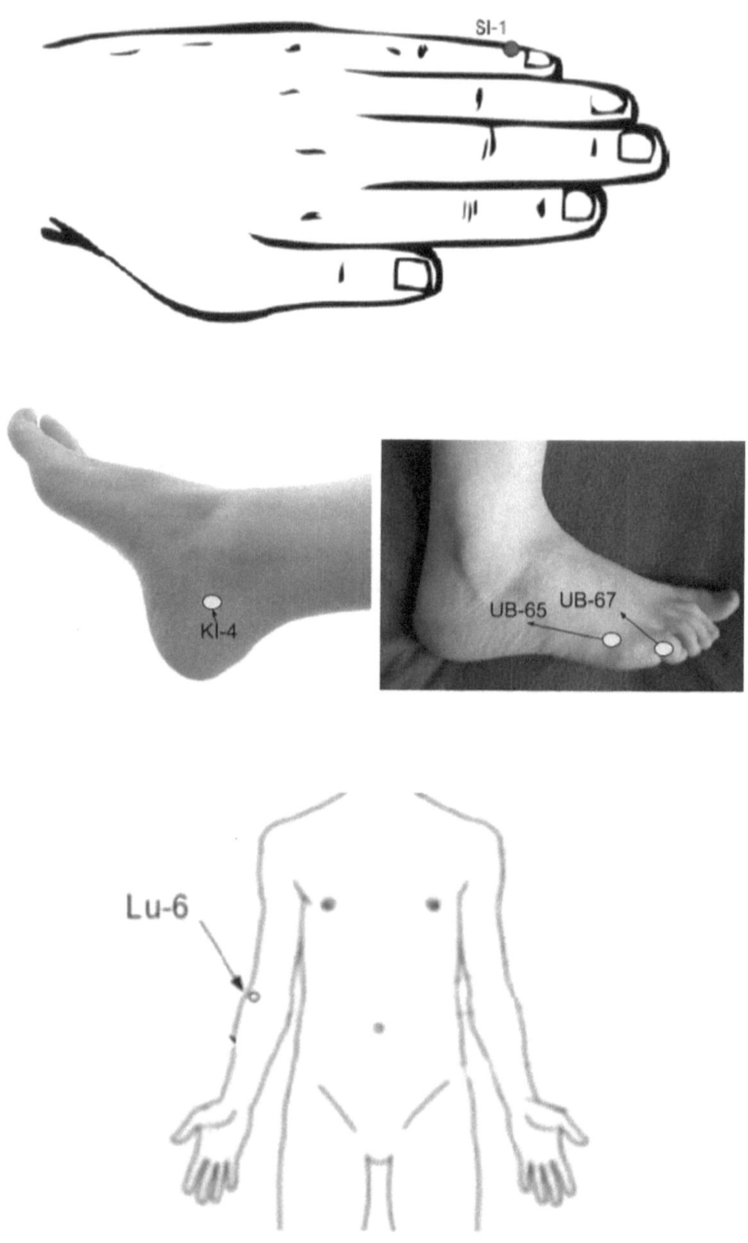

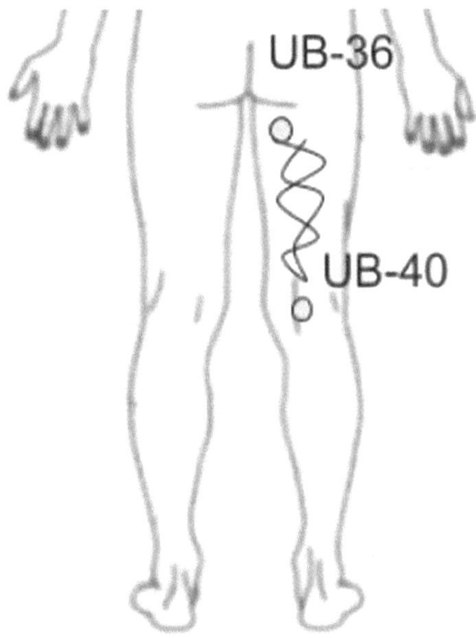

Other treatments for hamstring strains

Acupuncture is a very common treatment for hamstring strains, as is regular massage and moxibustion. To prevent blood stagnation, use herbs like myrrh, frankincense, black catechu, and more. Therapists might recommend blends like safflower and peach seed, which makes Tao Hong Si Wu Tang. There are herbal drinks that encourage good circulation, too. If there's swelling, anti-inflammatory herbs and food are also helpful.

Shin splints

Officially known as medial tibial stress syndrome, shin splints occur in runners, tennis players, dancers, soccer players, and any other athletes who use their legs a lot. It happens because the athlete is doing too much too soon. They aren't stretching well enough, their shoes are worn, or they're favoring their dominant leg too much. That's the leg that will hurt the most. You'll experience shin splints on the inside of the shin, which is the medial area. You can also have anterior shin splints, which is more on the outside of the leg. Lift your foot up at the ankle and flex the foot - if you feel a lot of pain, you probably have shin splints.

What points should you target?

For a cupping massage, oil the side of your shin that has pain. Place the cup just under the knee and massage down to your ankle. Massage up and down for 2-4 minutes at least once a day.

There are two specific pressure points you can target for shin splints. Apply cups on ST-36 and ST-39 on the leg that hurts, and maintain suction for at least 5 minutes. For best results, do this twice a week for two weeks.

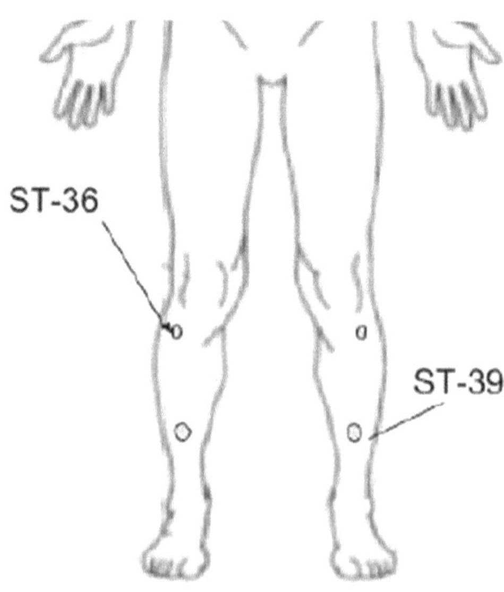

Other treatments for shin splints

Acupuncture and moxibustion are both practiced for shin splints. Your diet can also have a positive effect. Stock up on foods high in calcium, vitamin K-2, and vitamin D. This includes raw nuts, bananas, kale, and avocado. For herbs, there are lotions and salves made with ingredients like black peach, rhubarb, and Chinese foxglove root. When rubbed into your shins, they reduce inflammation, treat bruises, and stimulate good circulation.

Knee injuries

Knee injuries are extremely common for all sorts of athletes. Of these injuries, ligament and meniscus tears occur the most. Ligament tears in the knee occur when the tissues stretch too far or actually snap. Meniscus injuries are when the cartilage that stabilizes the knee joint and cushions it gets damaged or ripped. Specific injuries include:

> **ACL (anterior cruciate ligament) injury** - the tissue band inside your knee joint stretches or tears.
>
> **PCL (posterior cruciate ligament) injury** - occurs when the ligament behind the ACL stretches or tears.
>
> **MCL (medial collateral ligament injury** - ligament on outside of kneecap that connects thigh bone to shinbone stretches or tears.
>
> **LCL (lateral collateral ligament)** - ligament on opposite side of the MCL stretches or tears.
>
> **IT band syndrome (Iliotibial band syndrome)** - an overuse injury affecting the ligament on outer part of thigh from the hip down to the shin.

Athletes who run a lot, repeat the same motions, and fall,end up hurting their knees frequently, though you can also get injured by riding a bike or kneeling for long periods of time. IT band syndrome is the most common overuse injury for runners. Symptoms of knee injury include pain, swelling, stiffness, redness, excessive warmth, weakness, and an inability to straighten your knee.

What points should you target?

There are lots of pressure points a therapist can use to treat a knee injury. To reduce tension and swelling, SP-9 is good, though it may be tender. LV-8 is another point that can reduce swelling. If you have problems with your meniscus, ST-35 and extra point Ex-LE-5 can be stimulated. This pair of extra points is known as "the eye of the knee." On the graphic, you can see the point that's on the inside side of the leg. The other one is parallel to it right on the outside of the knee in the little groove under the bony cap of the knee that sticks out when bent.

For generalized tendon healing and to reduce stiffness, cupping GB-34 can help, which you can find on the outside of your leg. Since IT band syndrome causes pain on the outside of the leg, this is a good place to cup for that condition. If it's too tender, use light cupping or acupressure. For tension around your knee, cup UB-39.

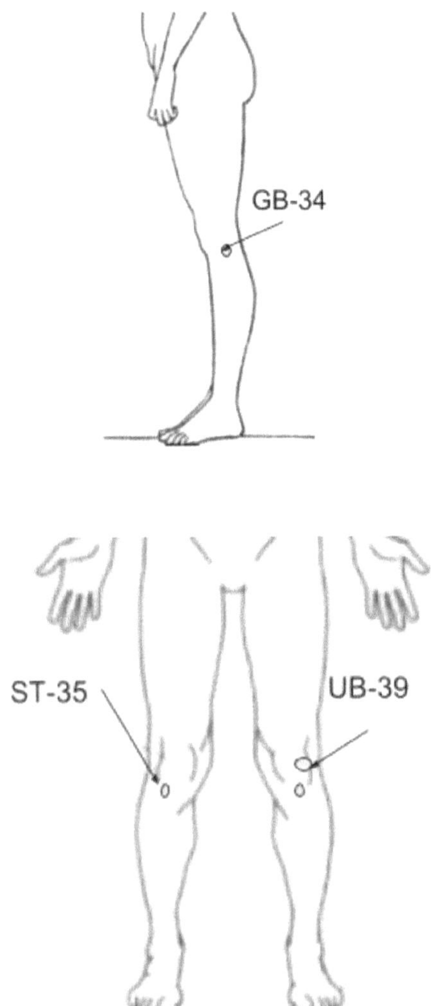
GB-34
ST-35
UB-39

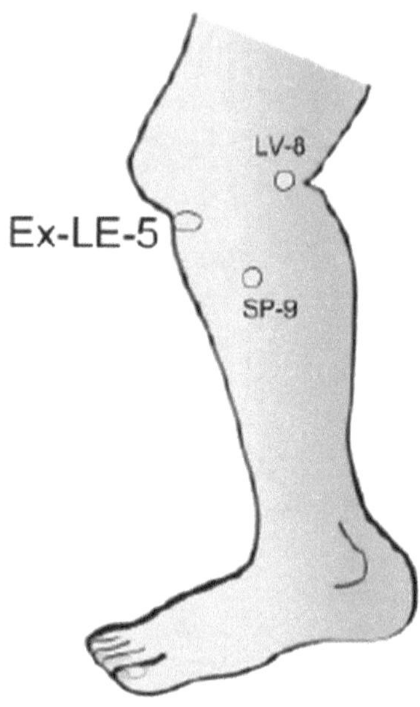

Other treatments for knee injuries

Acupuncture is a very common treatment for knee injuries. Like cupping, it relieves pain and encourages the body to heal faster. For diet, start eating more foods rich in vitamins like zinc, vitamin C, and vitamin D. Chicken, whole grains, nuts, kale, and berries are all good choices. Keep exercising (assuming you haven't torn anything), but don't do anything high-impact that stresses the injury. You just want to keep moving to prevent blood stagnation and stiffness. If you're looking for herbs, check out blends that include angelica, safflower, licorice root, and so on.

Tennis elbow

When your elbow tendons swell, you get tendinitis. That swelling is caused by forearm muscle overuse, and the pain occurs in the elbow and arm. The tendons connect your lower arm to the bone and repetitive gripping activities, especially those that use the ring and middle fingers and the thumb, cause inflammation.

Tennis, racquetball, and squash players can get tennis elbow, as can weightlifters and fencers. Symptoms of tennis elbow include pain on the outside of your elbow and when you move your wrist or grip. The pain radiates from the outside of your elbow to your forearms, and weakens you. Tennis elbow will also make your elbow feel stiff, especially in the morning.

What points should you target?

Two large-intestine points are effective for treating elbow pain. Cup LI-1 and LI-5, which are on the hand.

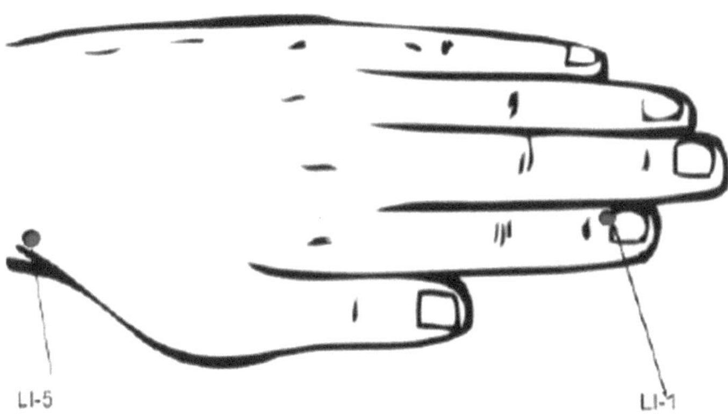

TB-6 and TB-10 are points especially good for tennis elbow. These triple burner (or triple warmer or triple heater) points do not correspond to any organs. They are a special meridian. TB-10 is also known as the "heavenly well," and is found in the depression about one's thumb length above (moving up your upper arm, not your forearm) the bony tip of the elbow when you have the elbow flexed. You can also cup LU-5 and LU-6.

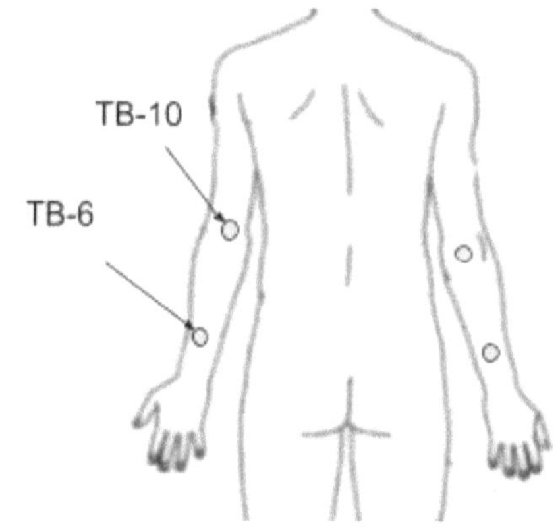

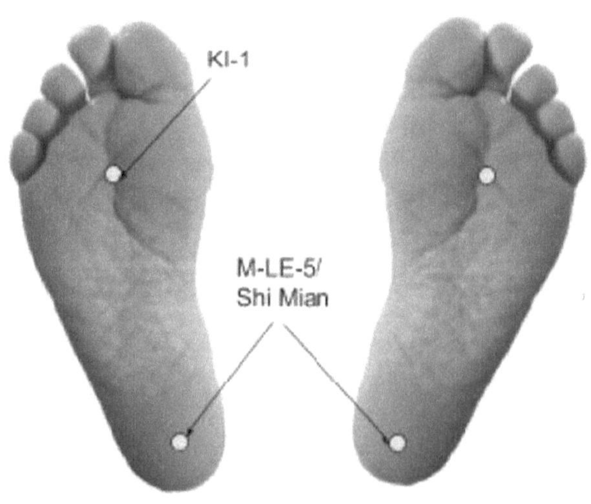

Other treatments for tennis elbow

Therapists use acupuncture as well as cupping to help tennis elbow. They will also likely have you engage in stretching exercises to keep blood circulating and stiffness at bay. To fight inflammation, you can change your diet and add more known anti-inflammatories like dark leafy greens, berries, and foods with magnesium. Cypress, peppermint, and frankincense can reduce pain and speed up healing.

Summary

You now know how to treat the six most common sports injuries using cupping. Areas on your hands and feet will require small cups, while wider, flatter areas like your back usually need larger cups. Some points are so small - like the ones on your fingers - you will probably just be able to apply acupressure instead of cupping. To enhance the cupping treatment, read the other treatment recommendations carefully. Following a healthy diet with herbal formulations will only benefit you and can strengthen your body against further injury.

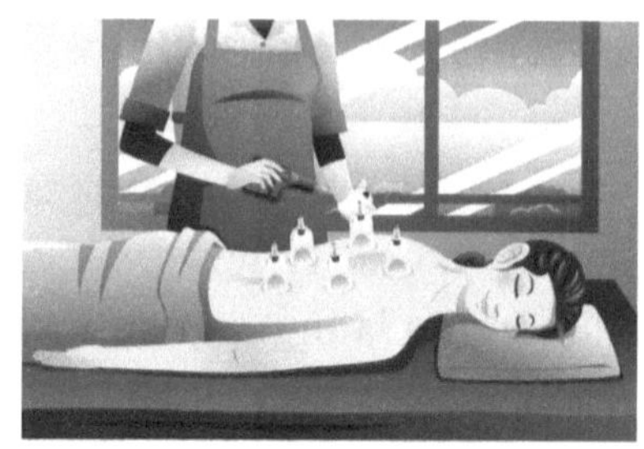

C h a p t e r   6

Guides for Other Injuries

Athletes can fall victim to many other injuries besides the most common we just discussed. Some arise as a result of one of those injuries while others develop on their own. In this chapter, we'll cover more injuries athletes might experience, beginning at the feet and working our way up. These guides are meant for educational purposes only and do not replace actual medical advice. If you believe you might have one or more of the conditions listed, please see your doctor.

Plantar fasciitis

Caused by an inflammation of the plantar fascia, the connective tissue supporting the arch of the foot, plantar fasciitis is the most common cause of heel pain for athletes. Just about every sport experiences it, while even just walking and standing on a hard surface for a long period of time can cause it. Studies have shown that dry cupping can relieve pain caused by this condition. It's especially effective when combined with electrical stimulation therapy like electroacupuncture.

What points should you target?

There are several points you can cup to treat plantar fasciitis. The first is a distal point located in the hand. It's known as Shaofu HE-8. You'll use a small cup for this area. Other points you can cup include KI-4 and KI-5, and KI-7 and KI-8. Cup these in pairs, since stimulated together, they increase the cupping's effectiveness.

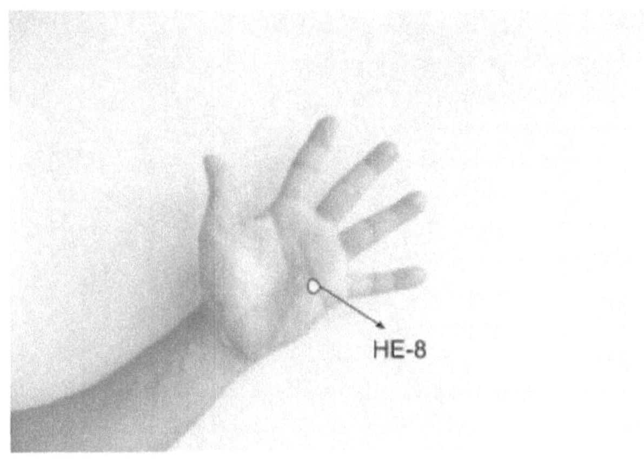

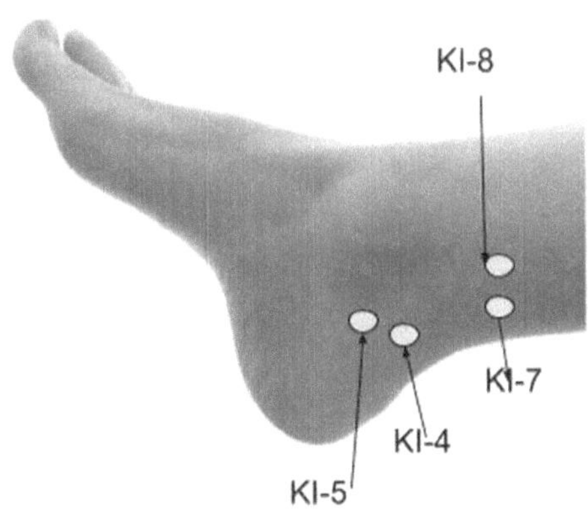

Cupping these areas before you treat the actual area of injury can help reduce discomfort. KI-1 is right in the plantar fascia, and it's known as Yongquan, "The Gushing Spring." Cupping it with LV-3 improves ligament and tendon health. The point known as M-LE-5, however, is known as an "extra point." Known as Shi Mian or Shimian. It's considered "extra" because in World Health Organization's 1991 report listing acupuncture points, they named 361 acupuncture points, and then 48 "extra" ones. You can find the Shi Mian point in the center of your heel.

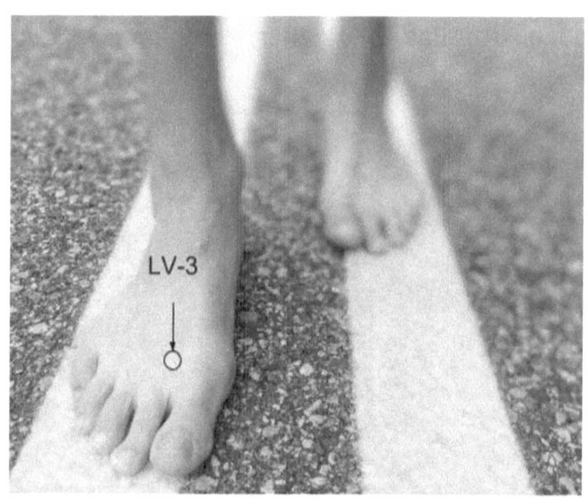

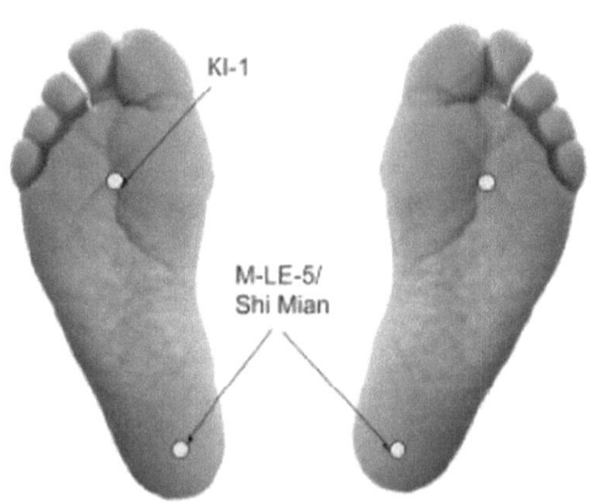

Other treatments for plantar fasciitis

Therapists often use acupuncture for this foot condition, specifically by inserting needles right into and around the Shi Mian points. As you read, the pressure points targeted are all kidney or liver meridians. That means those organs are both being affected and affecting the foot pain. Eating foods that improve the health of those organs can help the foot pain, such as apples, sweet potatoes, and eggs. Avoid caffeine, sugar, and strong spices.

Achilles tendonitis

The Achilles tendon consists of a band of tissue connecting your calf muscles at the back of your lower leg to the heel bone. It's the largest tendon in the body. Tendinitis of the area occurs when it is overused. It's most common in athletes who increase the intensity or length of their workouts, and they aren't ready or don't prepare properly before a session. You'll also see Achilles tendonitis in casual basketball and tennis players. The tendon can even rupture or tear when the athlete jumps or pushes off. It's actually the most commonly-injured tendon. When the tendon tears, surgery is usually required, and then you can consider cupping.

Symptoms include swelling and pain in your heel during exercise. You'll also likely experience tight calf muscles and limited motion when you try to flex your foot. The skin on your heel might even feel warm.

What points should you target?

The tendon itself might be too tender to cup, but massage cupping anywhere around UB-57 to your calcaneus, which is the large heel bone, is acceptable. You can also use the extra M-LE-5 point we discussed in the plantar fasciitis section above. Applying light cupping at first is the best idea, since many therapists might not even recommend cupping for Achilles tendonitis. It can be very painful depending on how severe it is. Cupping should *not* be done if the tendon has actually ruptured.

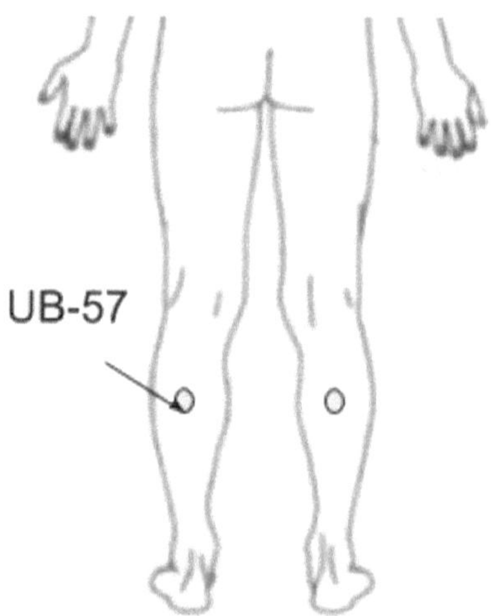

Other treatments for Achilles tendonitis

Massage therapy is the preferred method for treating tendonitis in the Achilles. It encourages blood flow and flushes out toxins without risk of damaging the tissue and tendon further. Therapists might also use acupuncture, and they will likely insert needles around the tendon to reduce inflammation. Stretching and moving the tendon is recommended to help with mobility and get the blood flowing to the injured area. Herb formulations will include ingredients like white peony, angelica, safflower, licorice root, and myrrh.

General foot pain

Foot pain is very common even if it isn't always as serious as plantar fasciitis or tendonitis. When your feet hurt, your whole body can start hurting, as well. Cupping the feet can improve your blood circulation and provide relief from stiffness and pain. General guidelines for foot cupping include cupping on the fleshiest parts and never cupping over an artery or a bone. Small cups are sometimes necessary, so you can get between bony areas.

What points should you target?

To treat foot pain, you can cup on the legs, since all those muscles are connected. UB-57 and UB-58 are common areas, as well as LV-1 (though you may have to just perform acupressure) and LV-3. KI-1 is the only acupuncture point on the soles of the feet, and is considered so important because it's where our bodies meet the earth. Yin is drawn up into the body through KI-1 while Yang descends.

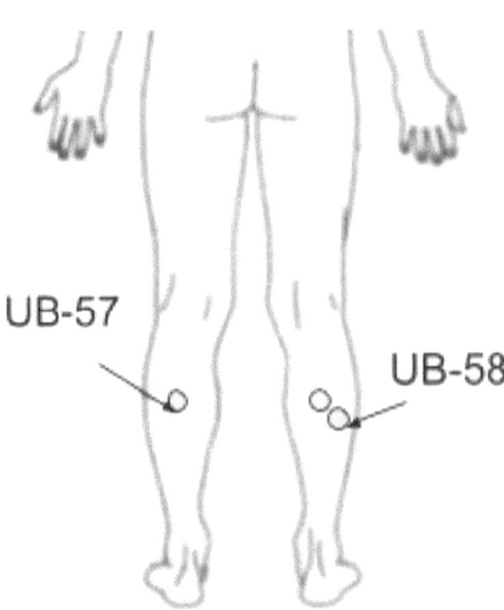

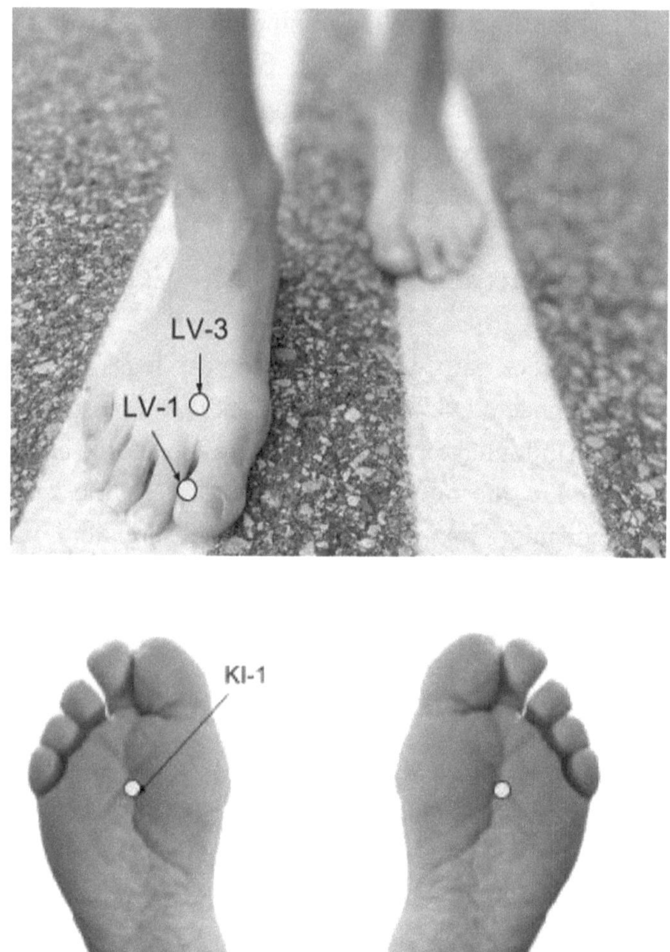

Other treatments for general foot pain

Generalized foot pain is more often than not caused by overuse. One of the best medicines is rest and relaxation. A warm foot bath with epsom salt can help, while some even swear by foot baths with peppermint or chamomile tea. You can also prevent foot pain by wearing shoes with thick, shock-absorbing soles.

Groin/hip pain

Oftentimes, your groin pain affects your hips and vice versa. Pain in this area makes it hard to do just about anything, let alone work out or engage in competition. Hip pain can occur after overworking the muscles or falling at a strange angle. Slipped capital femoral epiphysis is when the ball-and-socket hip joint becomes detached. Basically, the ball "slips off" the socket. It can happen suddenly when you fall or slowly over time. Pain can occur in both or just one hip, and it's usually within the groin or outside part of your hip. You might feel the pain down your thigh to your knee as well. This condition is treated with surgery, but cupping can be used during the rehab process.

What points should you target?

The pressure points found on the lower back (UB-23 through UB-35) can receive a cupping massage or stationary cupping, followed by moxibustion. This will open up the bladder meridian and encourage good circulation. UB-48 can be cupped, though it may be tender, so be cautious.

GB-29, 30, 31, and 34 are also great points to cup. They relieve pain, inflammation, tightness, and numbness.

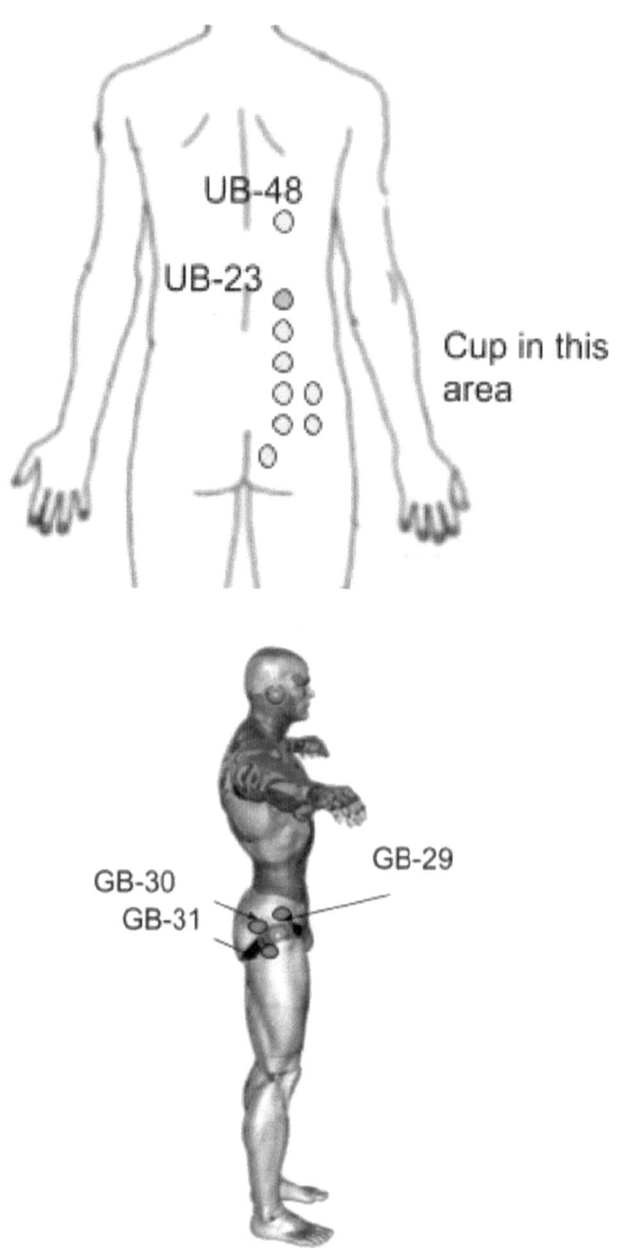

UB-48
UB-23
Cup in this area
GB-29
GB-30
GB-31

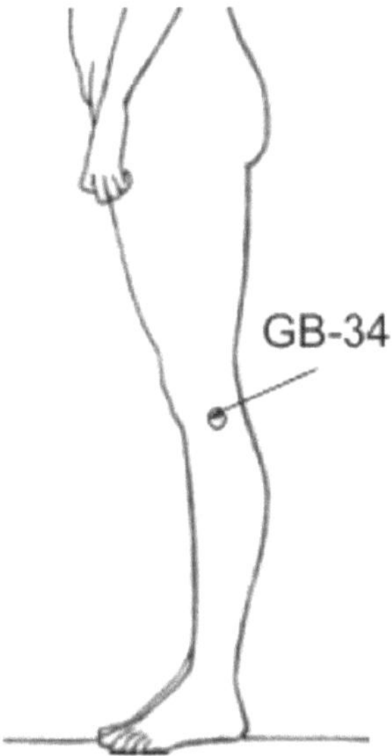

Other treatments for groin/hip pain

Soaking in a bath with epsom salts relieves sore and aching joints. You also want to keep moving, though not in a way that brings pain or discomfort. Be cautious and pay special attention to your form and posture. It's also a good idea to eat more anti-inflammatories like green tea, strawberries, ginger, blueberries, and spinach. Herbs like safflower, myrrh, and frankincense are also helpful.

Sports hernia

There are a variety of hernias, but the type that occurs in athletes is simply groin pain. The soft tissue (muscle, tendon, and ligament) in the lower abdomen or groin area becomes injured, causing tenderness and pain. It might even tear. Athletes who make quick changes in direction or twisting movements are the most vulnerable. Athletes with a "sports hernia" may not have a traditional hernia, so therapists will usually call the injury "athletic pubalgia."

Symptoms include immediate and severe pain upon injury. It will get better once you rest, but the pain returns when you go back to your sport. Twisting is especially painful. You *won't* see a bulge like you do with traditional hernias, though with time, an untreated sports hernia can result in the injured tissue forming a visible bulge.

What points should you target?

The therapist will determine the best treatment based on the severity of your injury. ST-29 and ST-30 are both considered good pressure points for treating hernias. You can also cup on points associated with pain relief for general groin pain: GB-29, 30, 31, and 34.

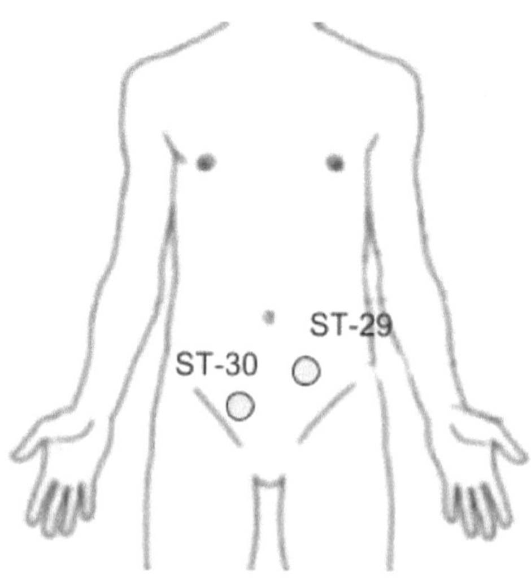

Other treatments for sports hernias

A 2-week rest is the best treatment for a sports hernia. The therapist will then begin physical therapy to help you regain strength and flexibility in your tissues, with cupping and acupuncture possibly playing a role at that time. Herbs like rosemary, thyme, and witch hazel can help with flexibility and increase your blood circulation. Look for formulations with these ingredients, as well as herbs that boost tendon and ligament health like safflower and peach seed.

Buttock pain

Sprinters and athletes who kick experience buttock pain, which may also extend to the lower back and thigh. There are a lot of joints and tendons in that area, including the hamstring and lumbar spine. Symptoms can include stiffness, muscle spasms, cramps, and pain.

What point should you target?

If you only feel pain in your butt, you can stationary cup with a medium to strong suction on UB-28, UB-54, and GB-30. If the pain extends into your legs and/or lower back, you can massage cup in the area by following your gluteus maximus muscle.

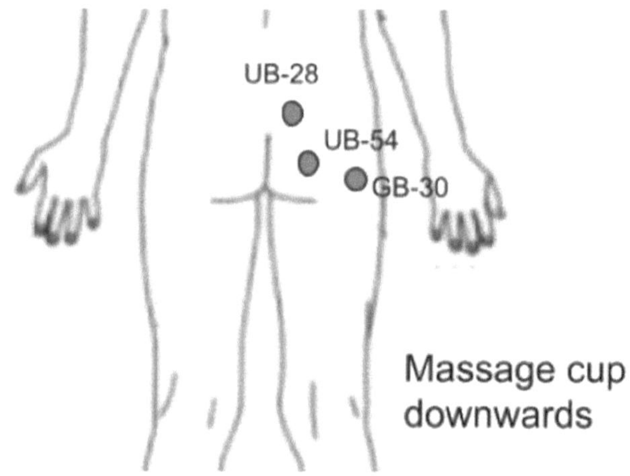

Other treatments for buttock pain

Massage and acupuncture are both employed for butt pain, along with cupping. Since therapists determined that a lot of this pain is caused by cold, they might also apply moxibustion to warm up the area. Electroacupuncture might also be used. For treatment at home, gentle stretching and rolling on a tennis ball can help keep blood circulating. Herb formulations will include ingredients like safflower, myrrh, red peony, and more. The goal is to encourage circulation, relieve pain and stiffness, and drive out cold.

Lower back pain

Lower back pain can happen to any athlete. It can occur suddenly or over time, and like all strains, it ranges from minor to severe. A strain happens when the muscle is stretched too far and becomes damaged or torn, while a *sprain* happens when the ligament is damaged. Ligaments keep the bones together. You can injure your lower back by lifting something heavy and twisting, getting hit hard in a sport, falling hard, or by having bad posture.

Symptoms include a dull, aching pain, as opposed to a sharp or burning feeling. You might also experience muscle spasms and aches in your hips and pelvis. If you have a tingling or numb pain in your lower back that extends to the buttocks, legs, and feet, you might have sciatica. This is usually felt on just one side of the body.

Lower back pain often becomes worse after you've been sitting for a while or asleep, and once you get moving again, it gets better. Certain positions can also be more comfortable than others. Therapists will use this information to figure out where the source of the problem is.

Bulging/herniated discs

Lower back pain can be caused by a bulging disc, which is when the inner part of a spinal disc swells through a space in the spine, past where it normally lies. This causes the "bulge." If there is no rupture or tear, you have a bulging disc, but if there is a tear, the gel-like nucleus actually *leaks* into the spinal canal. This means the disc has herniated or slipped. Bulging and herniated discs can occur anywhere in the spine, but about 90% of them occur in the lumbar/lower back area.

Athletes engaging in sports like running, weightlifting, football, and other sports that involve quick turns are vulnerable to disc injuries. Both bulging and herniated discs can put pressure on the nerves around it, causing pain. Sometimes, however, an athlete won't feel significant pain, so they don't know there's a problem.

What points to target?

The most effective pressure points depend on the type of back pain you have. For lower pain that's isolated just in the lower back, UB-26, UB-28, and GV-3 are good. If the pain radiates towards your buttocks, apply light cupping at UB-53, UB-54, and GV-3. UB-54, which you can find on both legs, relieves pain and stiffness caused by conditions like sciatica and herniated discs. It can also help knee and leg pain, stiffness, and muscle spasms.

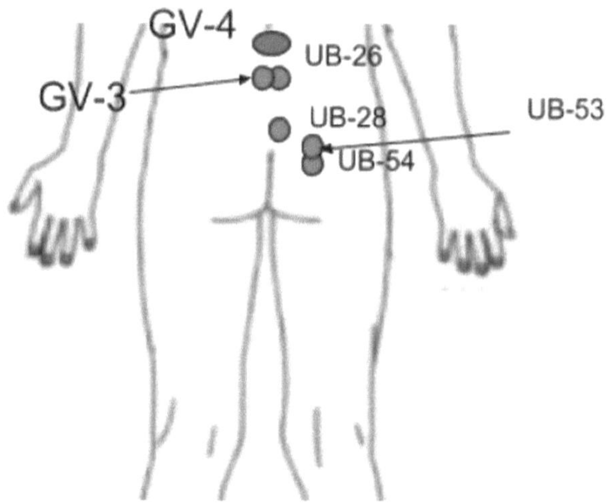

For pain on the lumbar spine (including bulging or herniated discs), cup UB-26, UB-28, and GV-3. The most effective pressure point for lumbar back pain, however, is GV-4, which is a Governing Vessel point. You can find it between the vertebrae at your waist in line with UB-23. GV-4 is also known as the "Life Gate" point.

For general lower back pain, there are more pressure points you can cup. UB-23 reduces muscle tension, while UB-47 specifically relieves tension in the quadratuslumborum muscles.

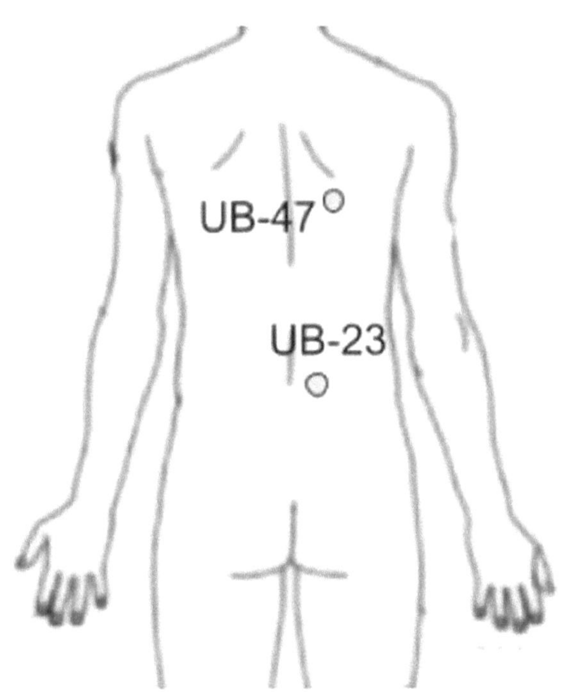

Other treatments for lower back pain

Acupuncture is a very common treatment for lower back pain. Like cupping, it relieves pain while encouraging proper blood circulation and healing. If you want to change your diet to decrease pain, stock up on anti-inflammatories like beets, carrots, sweet potatoes, cherries, and berries. Spices like basil, ginger, garlic, and rosemary are also known to reduce inflammation. In Traditional Chinese Medicine, the kidney and lower back are closely-related, so treating the kidneys can help relieve back pain. Herbs that encourage blood and qi flow are also good, such as red sage, turmeric, and safflower.

Cramps in the leg/ankle

Leg and ankle cramping can be simply annoying, or really painful and persistent. They are defined as contractions of the leg muscles and are often experienced when you're trying to sleep. They can be caused by conditions like dehydration, cold weather, poor blood flow, or overuse during exercise.

What points should you target?

There are several pressure points a therapist might cup. They will most likely first massage the points with the pads of their thumb to warm up the area. Cups will then be placed on ST-36 and SP-6. The bladder meridian is also important, so UB-40, 60, and 57 will be cupped for five minutes. UB-57 is known as the "Supporting Mountain" pressure point, and cupping it can relieve calf-muscle cramps, foot swelling, and knee pain. If your cramping is affecting your hips as well, UB-40 is a great point to stimulate. It's right at the back of the knee.

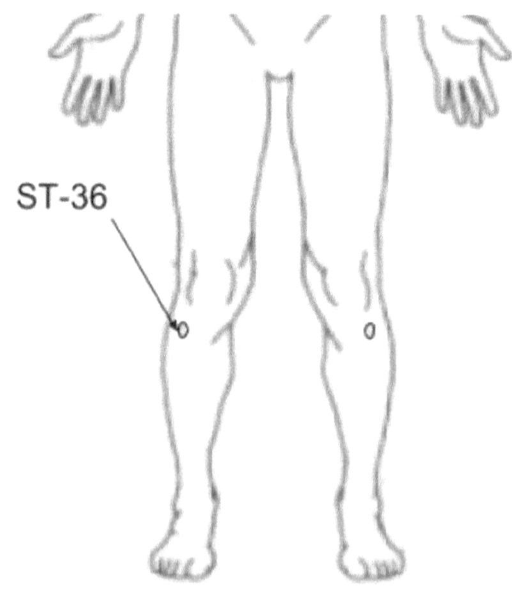

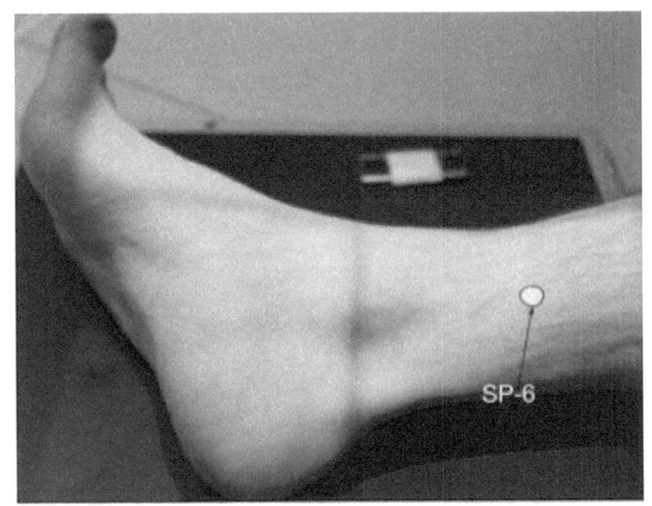
SP-6

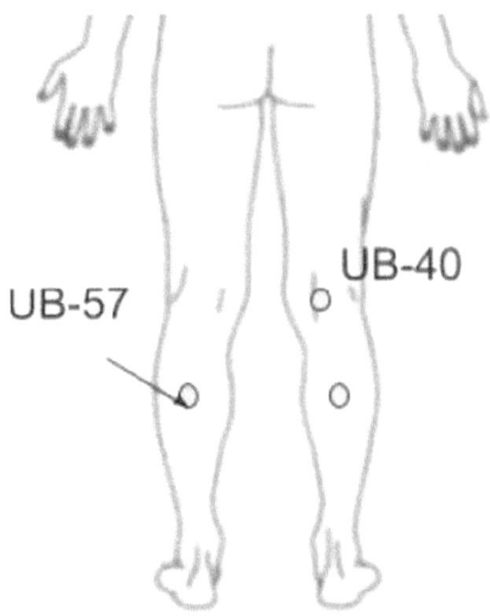
UB-40
UB-57

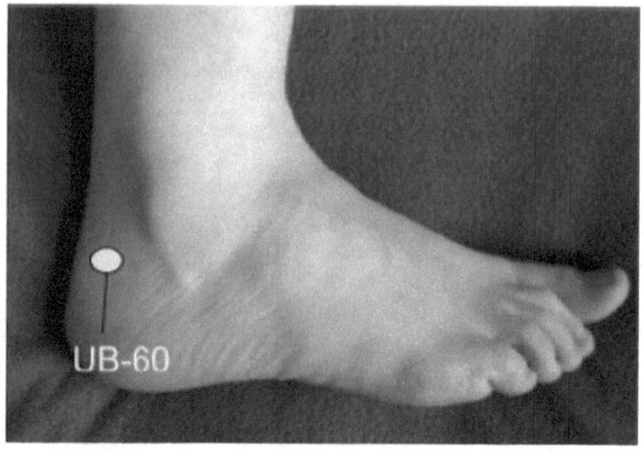

Other treatments for leg and ankle cramping

Cold causes a lot of cramping in the legs and ankles, so warming up the muscles before you work out is very important. You should also be sure to stay warm at night, especially if you're experiencing the cramping when you're trying to sleep. Stretch before bed to get the blood flowing. For food, get more calcium and potassium by eating dark-leafy greens, nuts, seeds, and bananas. As always, be sure to stay hydrated.

Varicosity

In addition to genetics, varicosity (varicose veins) can be caused by stress on the veins in your legs. High-impact sports like weightlifting, hiking, and skiing cause stress. Your muscles need more oxygen, which means increased blood flow through your veins. This can stress them out, causing them to swell and ache. Fatigue is another symptom. If untreated, varicosity can impact performance and training.

What points should you target?

Lung and blood health are the most important considerations in Traditional Chinese Medicine when it comes to varicosity. Improving their function improves the body's ability to carry oxygen-rich blood to the legs and everywhere else. Cupping can be performed on SI-14, UB-57, and SP-6. SP-10 is another significant point, and in Chinese, it's called the "sea of blood." It cools excess heat and plays a huge role in strengthening and moving blood. Hold the suction on these points for 5-10 minutes. A therapist might perform moxibustion afterwards.

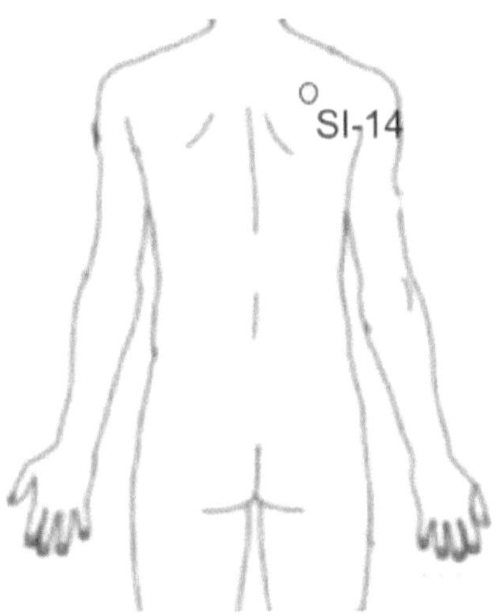

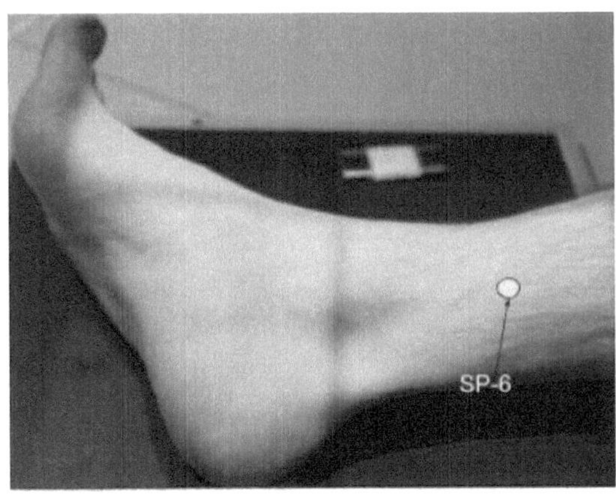

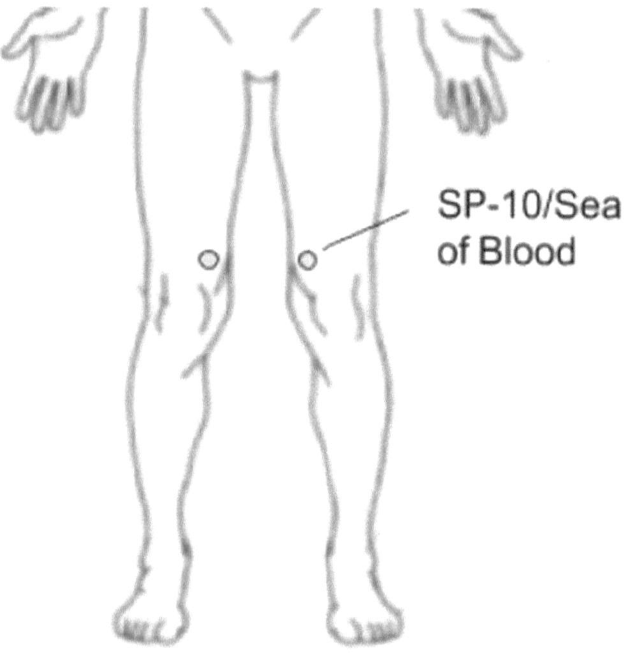

Other treatments for varicosity

Rest and hydration are easy, but essential treatments for varicosity. Avoid stressful training and standing too long. Since the spleen plays an important role in blood health, eat foods and herbs known to improve spleen qi. Grapes, sunflower seeds, sweet potatoes, ginger, brown rice, and horse chestnut are good choices.

Quad strain

The quad muscles are at the front of the thigh. They cross the hip and knee joints. They're essential for running, kicking, and jumping, so when they're injured, it's challenging to even walk properly. Like all strains, there are grades, with the 1st grade being a minor pulling that can be treated easily. The most serious strains are actual tears, and may require surgery. Football and rugby players experience quad injuries frequently.

Symptoms of quad strain include inflammation, swelling, and trouble straightening or bending your knee. When you try running, jumping, or kicking, you will feel pain. Your quads will also feel stiff and weak.

What points should you target?

You can cup the same points for quad strains as you did for hamstring strains. These are distal points that help heal the tendons: UB-65, UB-67, SI-1, LU-6, and KI-4. To see all those locations, read back to Chapter 5. For the actual injury area, apply light to medium massage cupping along the outside of the quad (the vastuslateralis) up to the middle of the top of the thigh (rectus femoris).

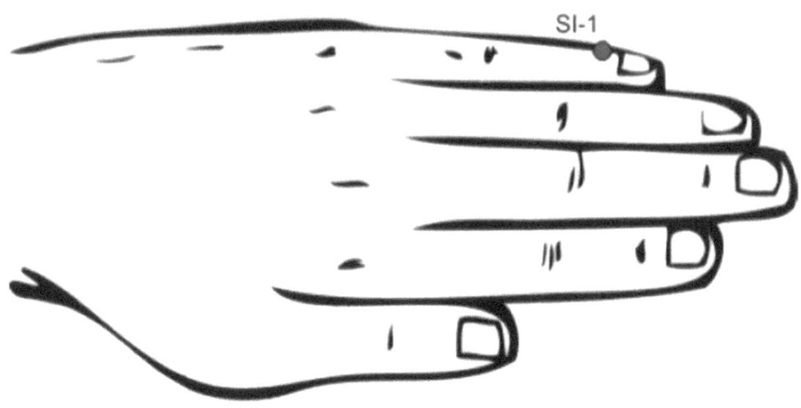

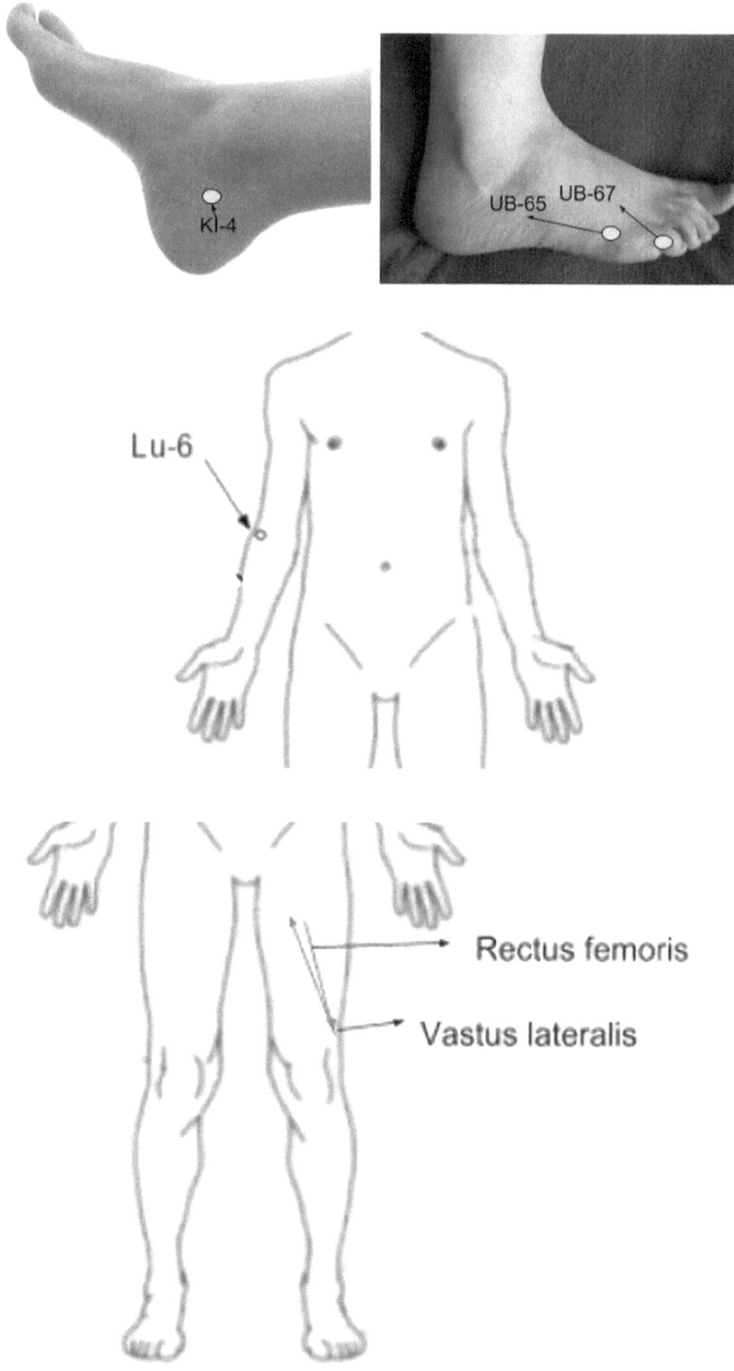
KI-4
UB-65
UB-67
Lu-6
Rectus femoris
Vastus lateralis

Other treatments for quad strains

Depending on how severe your strain is, your therapist might recommend a lot of rest. Careful stretching exercises can keep the blood moving, but you don't want to risk stretching the muscle further. Since the liver is in charge of strengthening tendons and ligaments, you want your treatment to target that organ. Eat a diet rich in liver-cleansing foods like seeds, fresh fruit, and vegetables, and drink plenty of water. Herbs like dandelion, angelica, ginger, and chamomile flowers can also strengthen the liver and ease inflammation.

Carpal tunnel syndrome

CTS is caused by an irritation of the median nerve. This is the nerve that runs from your forearm through a "tunnel" in your wrist to your hand. It's responsible for giving feeling to your thumb and all your fingers except the little one. If the median nerve becomes squeezed or irritated by an injury, you can develop CTS. Athletes who grip things (like cyclists, golfers, and tennis players) can get CTS.

CTS feels like a tingling pain in your hand and wrist. All your fingers except the little finger will also be affected. You might also feel numbness and weakness.

What points should you target?

There are quite a few points you can cup to provide relief and healing from CTS. Therapists will cup the large-intestine meridians LI-4, LI-5, and LI-10. On the wrist, they might also cup LU-8, which can help decrease numbness. PC-6 and TB-5 are also good points. Of TB-14 and LI-15, cup the place that's more tender.

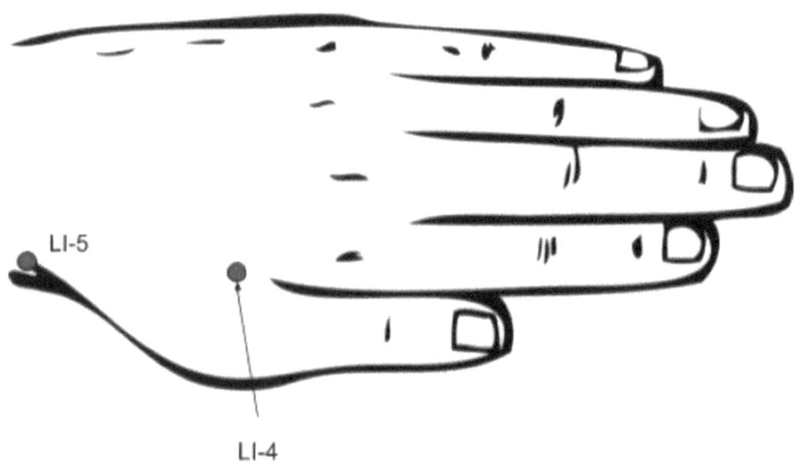

LI-5
LI-4

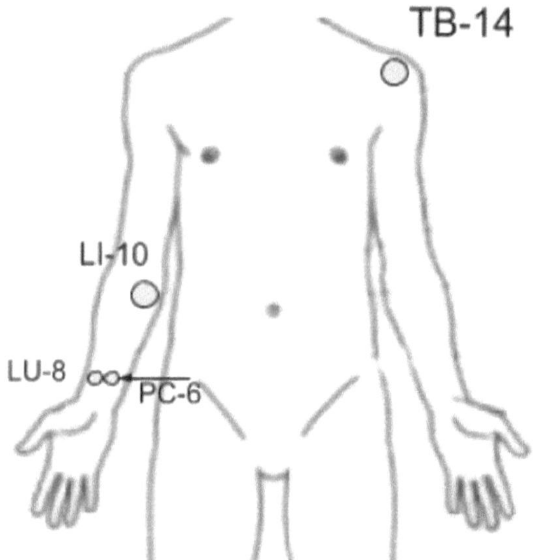

TB-14
LI-10
LU-8
PC-6

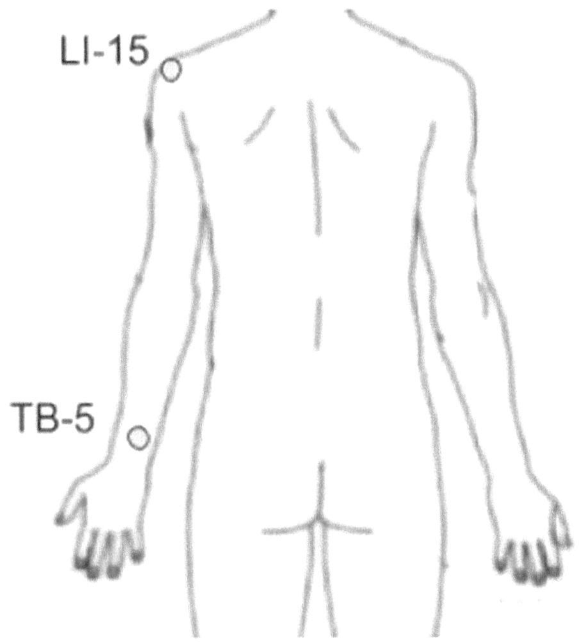

Other treatments for carpal tunnel syndrome

Acupuncture is a common treatment for CTS and has been shown in studies to relieve pain and possibly cure the condition. Therapists might also recommend splinting the wrist to keep it straight, especially at night, because this reduces pressure on the median nerves. You should also keep warm at night as cold aggravates CTS. Look for herbal formulations with ingredients like corydalis, a relative of the poppy that is very effective at reducing nerve pain. Foods rich in vitamin B6 and B12 can also help reduce inflammation, so eat up salmon, kale, strawberries, and spinach.

Wrist pain

Most athletes are at risk for a wrist fracture or sprain at some point in their lives. Fractures occur when you damage the long bones of your forearm or the smaller bones in the wrist. Falling on your outstretched hand can cause a fracture. Sprains, as we've mentioned before, are when the ligaments get injured. There are several in the wrist area because there are so many bones, and ligaments attach bone to bone. A sprain is less serious than a fracture.

You can sometimes tell the difference between a fracture versus a sprain by your symptoms. Sprains, which are less serious, actually hurt more. If you see that your wrist looks odd or that it appears the bone is poking out, it's a fracture. Both injuries cause swelling, bruising, weakness, and pain. You won't cup on a fracture, but you can cup its distal points to speed healing.

In addition to bone and ligament injuries, your wrist tendons can become damaged, too. There are several tendons that connect your hand muscles to your forearm. These are found in the wrist, and let the forearm muscles flex, extend, and wiggle your wrist. If you move your hand improperly, you can overwork the tendons, and they become inflamed. You'll experience swelling and pain, and it's hard to move your wrist.

What points should you target?

When cupping for pain relief from wrist injuries, there are five points a therapist might target. Two are Triple Burner points: TB-4 and TB-5. They can relieve pain and strengthen the wrist.

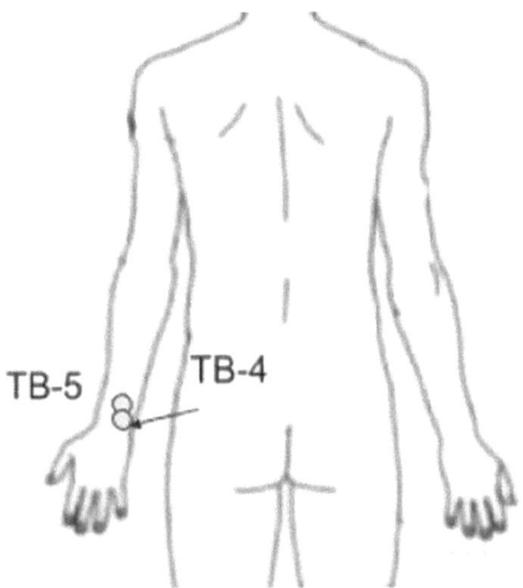

PC-6 and PC-7 can also be cupped. PC-7, on the Pericardium meridian, is especially effective at relieving pain in the wrist and thumb. The last point, LI-10, is good for wrist, elbow, and shoulder pain.

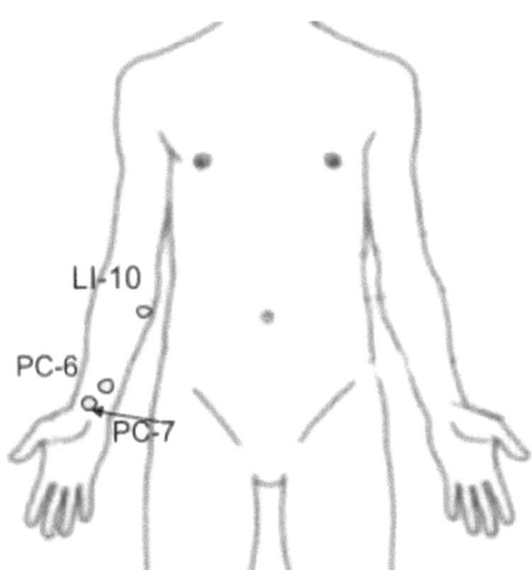

Other treatments for wrist pain

Acupuncture and electroacupuncture are very popular for wrist injuries and pain. Regular massage is also a common practice, since the hand may be too tender for cupping. If you have a lot of swelling, herbs like ginger can help. To boost your ligament and tendon strength, get formulations with peach seed, safflower, Himalayan teasel root, and cassia bark. Anything that relieves pain is good, too. Be sure to keep warm at night to prevent stiffness and blood stagnation.

Hand pain

There are a lot of small muscles, tendons, and soft tissue in your hands. These can become overstretched and fatigued, and nerves that extend into your arms can be affected. There's even a nerve root in your cervical spine that can cause pain in your hand and fingers when it comes compressed or irritated.

The hand can also develop tendinitis. De Quervain's Tendinitis occurs in the tendons in the thumb-side of your wrist. The lining or "sheath" of the two tendons responsible for controlling the thumb become inflamed. The sheath and tendons swell and irritate the nerves, triggering pain and numbness. It's sometimes called "Gamer's Thumb" or "Texting Thumb" because it's common among those who play a lot of video or computer games, and who hold their phone a lot.

Dupuytren's Contracture is most likely a genetic disease, and if you're an athlete who use your hand a lot, it can be a big problem. With this condition, the soft tissue on your palm thickens and contracts. You might feel small lumps in your palm that feel tender and painful, as well as cords of tissue that keep your fingers from spreading apart.

The last injury we'll cover is often known as "Skier's Thumb." The ulnar collateral ligament (UCL) is injured, commonly when a skier falls on their outstretched hand while gripping their pole. The soft tissue is damaged, and the UCL might be torn completely, separating the thumb for its normal place. Skier's Thumb can also happen while playing goalkeeper in soccer, wrestling, volleyball, or performing gymnastics. Surgery is often required to put the thumb back into place.

What points should you target?

The best points for cupping depend on what your primary hand issue is. One of the most effective points for hand pain in general is LI-4, which is on the back of your hand. You'll use very small cups for cupping on your hands. LI-11 is another good point, and it's on your elbow, so if your hand is too tender, choose this point instead of LI-4.

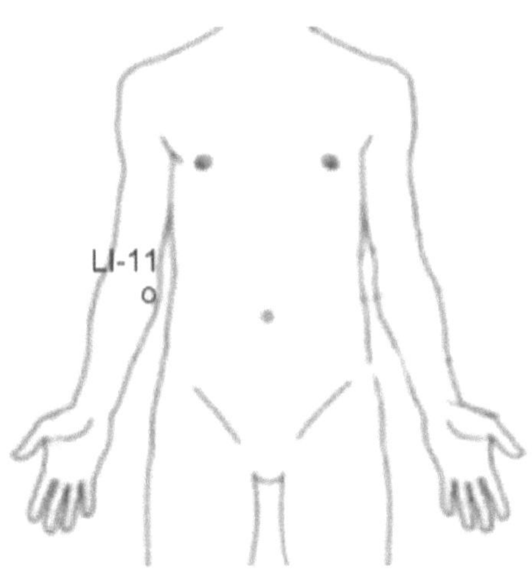

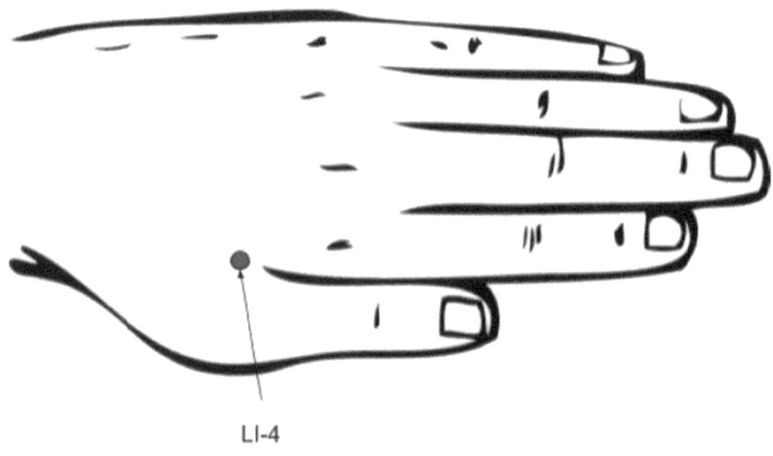

If you are experiencing a lot of hand numbness, stationary cupping LU-11, PC-8, and HE-3 can help. LU-11 is a very small point right by your thumbnail on the outside of your thumb. Apply acupressure if cupping is too tricky. HE-3 is very close to LI-11. If your grip is weak, SI-7, TB-4, and TB-10 can help you build up your strength.

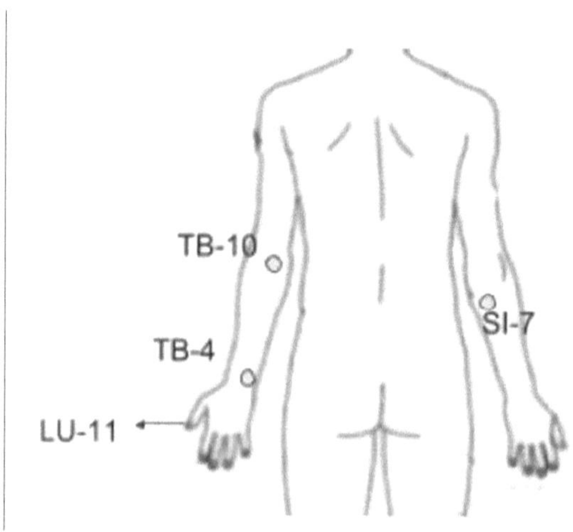

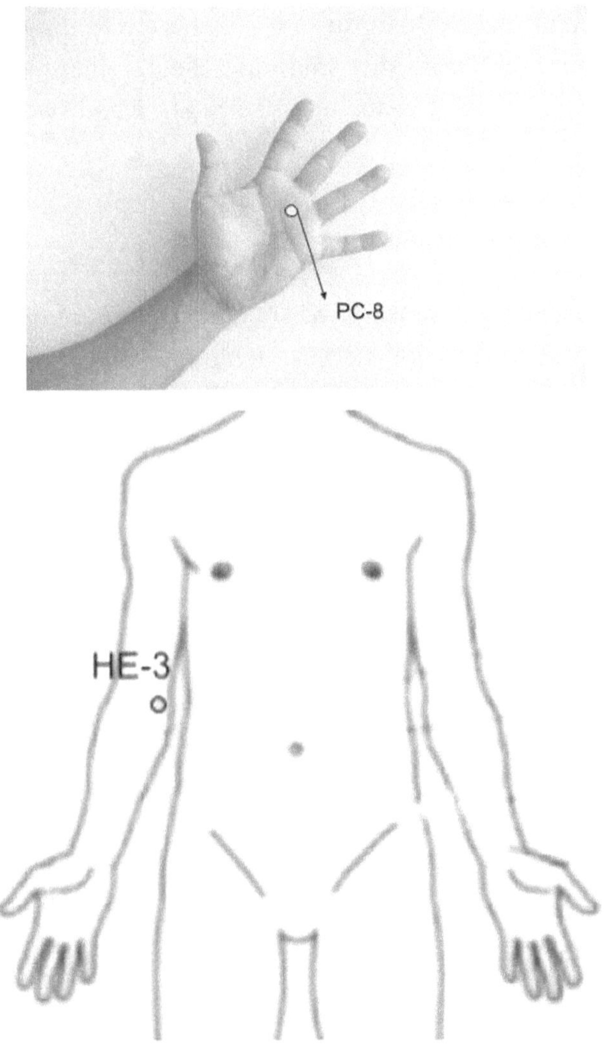

Other treatments for hand pain

Acupuncture is a common treatment for hand pain, as is regular massage. Therapists will also recommend gentle stretching exercises to prevent blood stagnation. If your hands hurt, try soaking them in hot water for 10-15 minutes. This improves circulation and relieves painful joints. A herb like the thunder god vine (Tripterygiumwilfordii) can also help, since it has been proven very effective at reducing inflammation and swelling.

Forearm pain

Hand, wrist, forearm, and shoulder pain are closely related since they share lots of nerves, tendons, and ligaments. The forearm is defined as the area between the wrist and elbow. We've discussed causes of arm pain already, like tennis elbow and carpal tunnel syndrome. Arthritis, broken bones, strains, sprains, and tendonitis can also cause pain.

A bad fall can cause injury on the forearm, as can overuse during sports that involve the arms a lot, like tennis and weightlifting. Symptoms can include numbness, shooting pain, and/or aching throughout your arms, wrists, and/or shoulder.

What points should you target?

LI-11 is also known as the "Pool at the Bend" and you can find it on the external side of the arm at the elbow. It can treat arm pain and inflammation, including symptoms of tennis elbow. PC-3 is another elbow point that relieves arm pain and tremors in both the arms and hands. LU-9 can be cupped with a small cup to treat arm and wrist pain.

A Triple Burner point can also help forearm pain. TB-14 is found on the shoulder. Cupping there can help with numbness and stiffness.

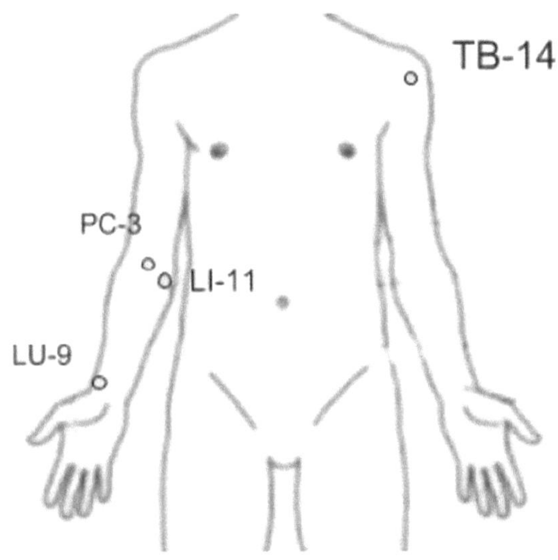

Other treatments for forearm pain

Acupuncture and massage therapy are both useful for treating forearm pain and bringing the patient back up to their regular strength. There are also elbow exercises and stretches a therapist might recommend. Rest, water, and plenty of food rich in zinc, vitamin D, and calcium ensure the proper healing process. For herbs, the thunder god vine, ginger, safflower, peach seed, and angelica boost tendon healing and strength.

Shoulder pain

Shoulder pain makes it hard to do anything. It can be caused by straining a muscle while engaging in a sport or doing heavy weight-lifting. The rest of your body is greatly affected, and even just lying down can be painful. Your shoulder has three bones, forming a ball-and-socket joint. The tissue that holds this joint together is called the shoulder capsule.

Pain that shoots down your arm might be caused by a rotator cuff injury. The rotator cuff (which is actually a bundle of four muscles sits atop your upper arm bone. An injury to this area starts out with a dull ache, but as soon as you move your arm, the pain sharpens. Athletes who engage in repetitive arm motions like baseball players and tennis are especially vulnerable.

"Frozen shoulder" is another common complaint, especially if you have diabetes or are older. What happens here is that the shoulder capsule actually thickens and becomes tight. Scar tissue builds up, and a fluid that keeps the joint nice and lubricated decreases. Shoulder movement becomes stiff and difficult.

What points should you target?

What pressure points are best can depend on where the pain is in your shoulder. If it's mostly in your shoulder joints, LU-2, LI-16, SP-20, SI-10, and TB-14 will be massaged well first. This warm-up is very important. Cupping can be applied for 15-20 minutes. If the pain is also in your arm, cup LI-14, LI-15, and TB-13. If the pain is located in the shoulder and neck, cup SI-12 and TB-15. Always massage with your hands first. After cupping, a therapist will likely perform moxibustion to enhance the cupping's healing power and ensure the shoulder stays warm as long as possible.

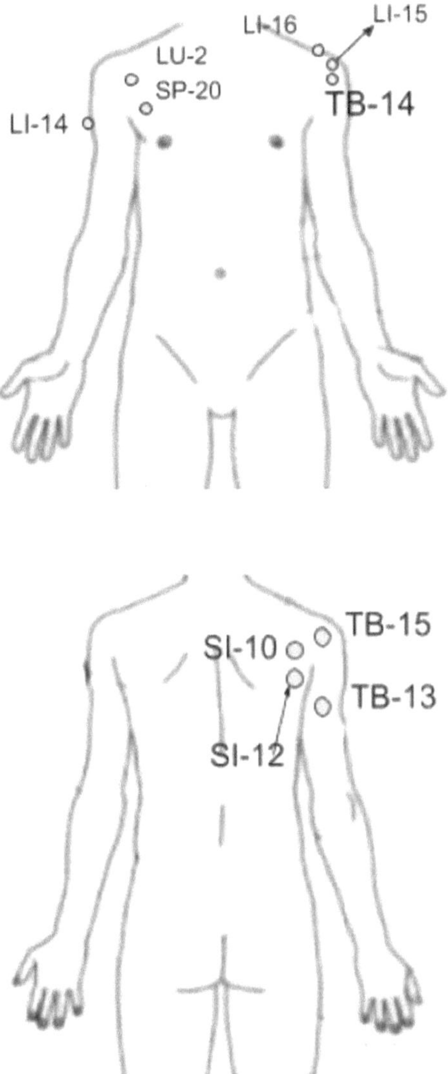

Other treatments for shoulder pain

Warmth is key when it comes to treating shoulder pain. Being cold will only increase the shoulder's stiffness and make recovery more challenging. Wear clothes that cover the area well, especially at night. You want to encourage good blood circulation. There are also herb formulations with ingredients like white peony, ginger, and angelica, which drive out cold and damp winds. Shoulder joint exercises are a good complement to cupping and acupuncture.

Neck pain

Your neck holds muscles and ligaments like the rest of your body, and these are vulnerable to strain. Sports that involve hitting and force (like football) can cause nerve damage, disc slips, strains, and more. Known as "burner" or "stinger" injuries, getting your head pushed to one side is a very common injury among football players. A bundle of nerves at this point becomes injured and can cause pain in your arm as well. When you're hit and your neck goes backward or forward, you can get a neck strain, which is often called whiplash. Like all strains, the force damages the muscles and tendons, while *sprains* injure the ligaments.

Cervical dislocation is a very serious neck injury. As ligaments are damaged, the neck bone actually moves from its normal position. In athletes, trauma usually causes this injury, and it often comes with a fracture. The ligaments can even rupture. Surgery is usually required. If the bone doesn't move all the way out of place, it can move back where it's supposed to be on its own if proper care is taken.

Symptoms of a serious neck injury include severe pain, a shooting pain in your arms and legs, numbness, tingling, and weakness. Neck strains feel like stiffness and tightness in your neck, pain when you try to move your neck back and forth (or side to side), tenderness, and headaches.

What points should you target?

Most of the points best for neck pain are actually on the head, which you cannot cup unless the patient is bald. UB-3 through UB-10 are all effective, and if you can't cup, you can apply acupressure to the points. The UB-3 through UB-8 points can be found on top of the head right where the forehead meets the top of your head, and along the left side moving towards the back of the head. UB-9 and UB-10 are at the back of the head.

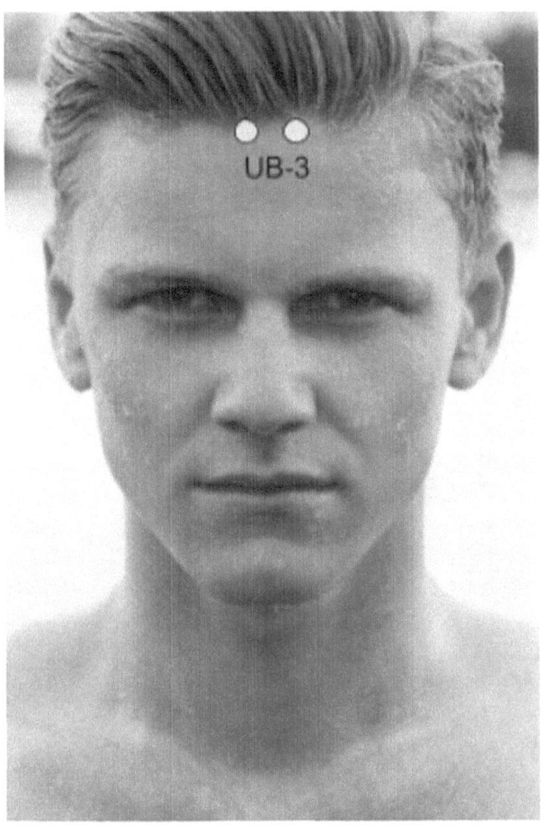

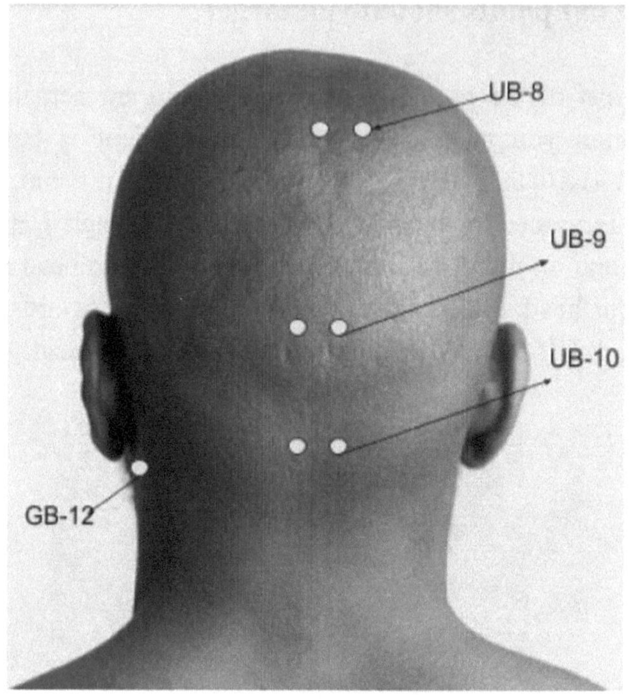

GB-12 and GB-21 are points you can cup and are probably hair-free. GB-12 is right under the earlobe and about a thumb's width toward the back of the head. GB-21 is on your shoulders.

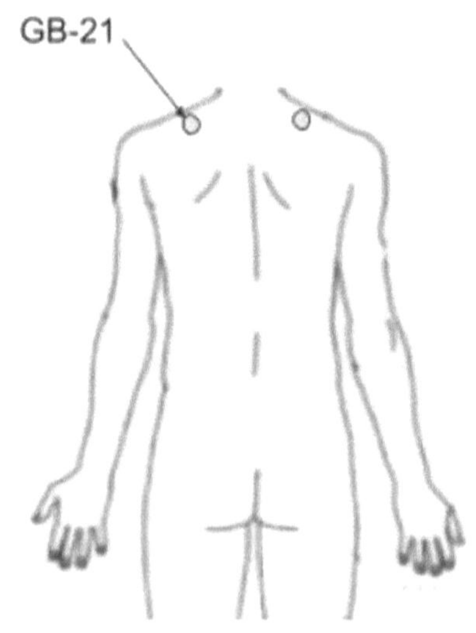

Other treatments for neck pain

Acupuncture and acupressure are popular for neck pain. Since many of the pressure points for neck pain are located on the scalp and head, acupuncture is practiced more frequently than cupping. In addition to massage and stretching, your diet can help relieve neck pain. Eat foods rich in anti-inflammatories, Vitamin C, and Vitamin D. For herbs, kudzu is used a lot in formulations (in both pill and powder form) for reducing inflammation. It does affect the body like estrogen. Other herbs include lavender, which helps relieve tension, astragalus, and Dangshen, also known as "poor man's ginseng."

Post-trauma headaches

After a concussion, an athlete might develop what's known as PTH or post-traumatic headache. It's common to experience headaches within a week of a head injury. The headache might be caused by a neck injury, inflammation, or nerve pain in the head. An athlete will feel a moderate to severe migraine with pulses. After a few months, the headaches usually should be gone, but if they aren't, it officially becomes PTH. Athletes who receive frequent blows to the head (football) are at risk for PTH.

Symptoms include pulsating pain in the head, dizziness, neck pain, headaches that get worse during workouts or mental exertion, concentration problems, insomnia, anxiety, and fatigue.

What points should you target?

The therapist will treat the areas of the face and head where you feel the pain radiating. They will use light cupping massage along the neck and flash cupping for the face, so marks don't appear. There are also distal points that can be effective, such as PC-6 and LI-4. GB-21 is another good point that can help relieve neck stiffness, as well.

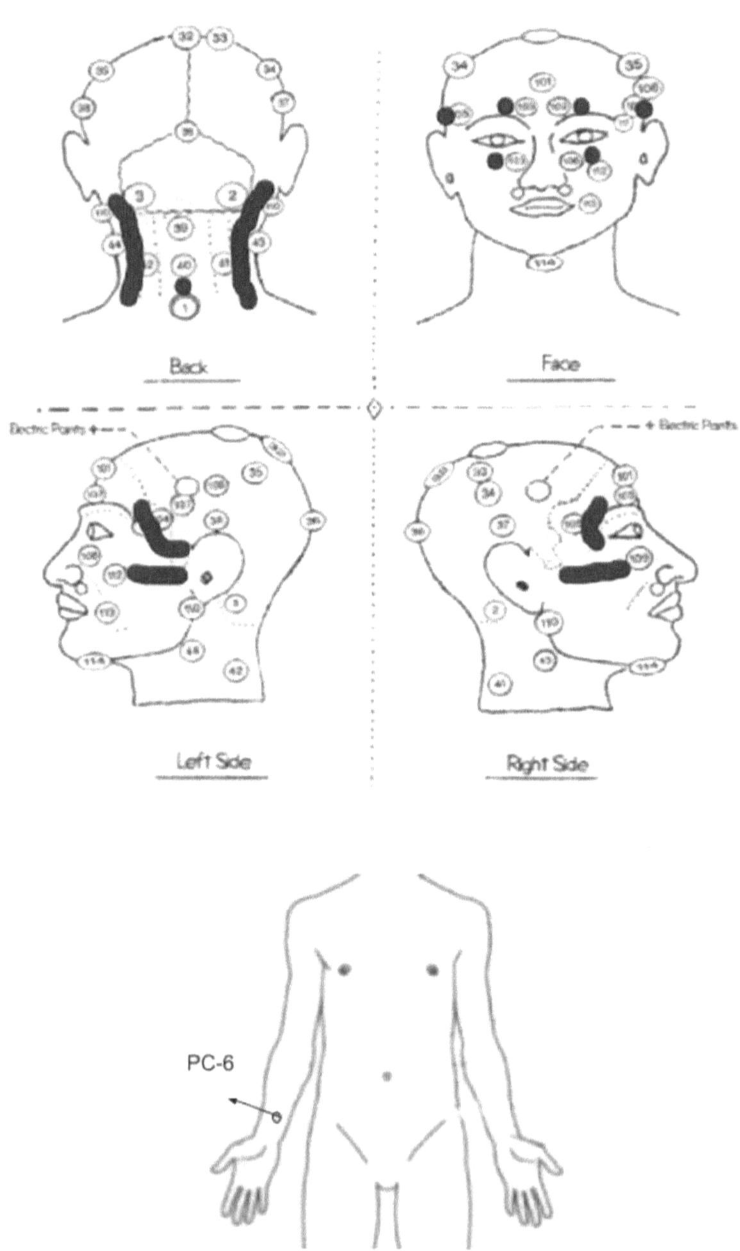

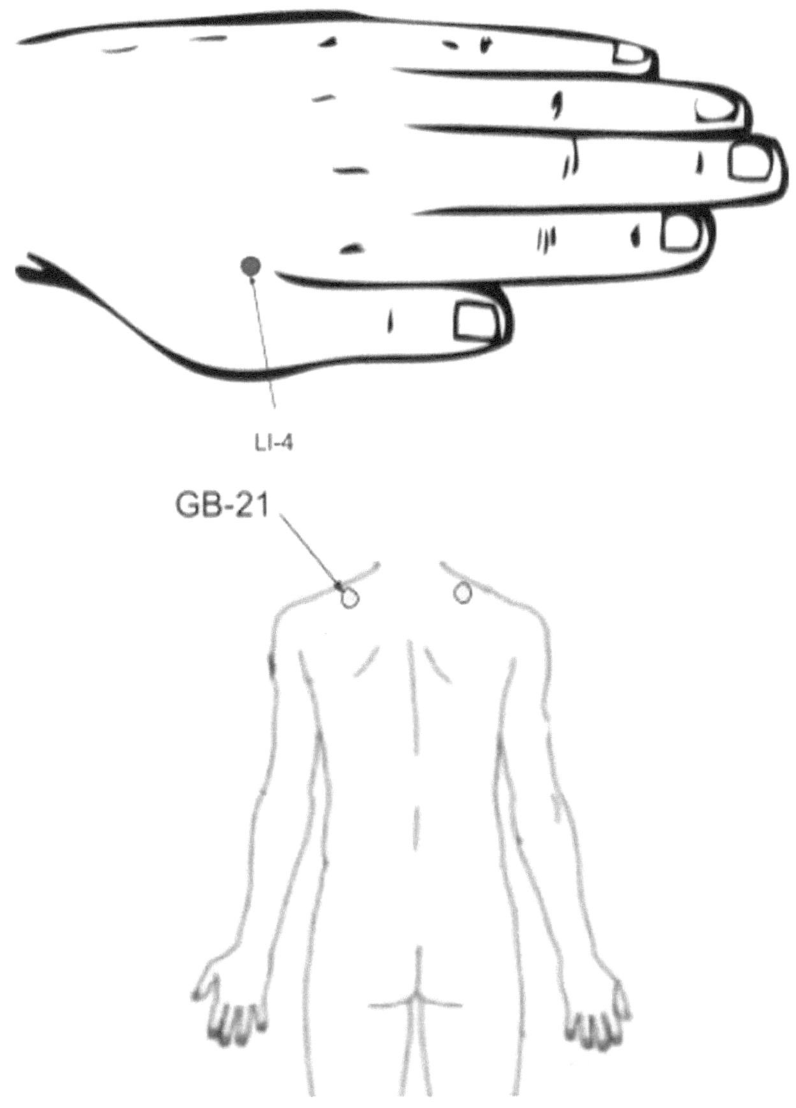

Other treatments for trauma headaches

Since trauma headaches can indicate a disruption in your brain's recovery process, it's very important to monitor them carefully. One of the best treatments is rest, both physical and mental. Take frequent breaks during work hours and avoid projects and activities that require a lot of concentration. Also avoid things that aggravate the headaches, like light, noise, certain food, and so on. A therapist might also recommend massage and/or acupuncture.

Stock up on healthy fats and foods rich in vitamin B12. It's also a good idea to eat frequently - every two hours or so - because your brain needs glucose in order to heal. Fruit is a good choice. For herbs, basil, chamomile, lavender, and wild ginger are all effective at treating headaches and encouraging relaxation.

Stress fractures

Stress fractures, also called "hairline" fractures, are tiny cracks in your bones. When you up the intensity of your workout, the bone's rebuilding process normally adapts and keeps up. However, if you increase your activity too much too soon, the bone tissue isn't able to rebuild quickly enough and teeny-tiny cracks form. Certain sports like basketball, tennis, dance, gymnastics, soccer, and track and field see a lot of stress fractures. The lower leg and foot are the most common places for this type of injury.

Stress fractures often start with little pain, but it gets worse as time goes on. You'll feel tenderness in the area, as well as swelling. The pain is usually deep and aching. It feels better with rest, but as soon as you start working out again, it comes back. Your performance might be affected. If the pain began after a change in your workouts, that's a sure sign it's a stress fracture.

What points should you target?

Cupping is actually *not recommended* for fractures. Acupuncture is used instead.

Other treatments for stress fractures

High-impact sports should be avoided during the treatment and healing process. However, movement is still a good idea because it encourages blood circulation and recovery. Swimming and cycling are often recommended. For your diet, increase your intake of minerals like zinc and calcium, since bones are about 70% minerals. Add more vitamin C, vitamin D, and vitamin B6, as well. Herbal treatments designed to relieve pain and encourage blood circulation can be included in your recovery plan. The herb eucommia, the bark from the Chinese rubber tree, is known for supporting bone and kidney health. Other herbs include red sage, astragalus, safflower, drynaria, dipsacus, teasel, and ginseng.

Adhesions/general stiffness

Cupping can be used when you haven't necessarily experienced a specific injury, but your legs are feeling sore and tense. This is especially common after you've healed from your injury and are getting back into your normal workout routines. During the healing process for sprains, tears, and breaks, scar tissue forms, and it becomes like knots under your skin. These are called "adhesions," and they occur when scar tissue binds tendons that aren't supposed to be together.

What points should you target?

You will massage cup on the affected areas. Instead of listing specific points, let's walk through the different techniques therapists might use. To begin, therapists warm the area well with a heating pad or 5 minutes of cardio. They will then apply a generous amount of oil.

The classic up-and-down massage is the most comfortable option, and is a good way to gauge how bad the adhesions are. Cross-fiber massage is when you move the cup side-to-side and up-and-down. It causes more discomfort as the cupping aims to break down the adhesions. If the area is swollen, red, or recently-injured, you shouldn't apply cupping. If the patient is in pain, stop. The last cupping massage is circular, and you apply it by moving the cup in circles on the soft tissue of the affected area.

Other treatments for adhesions

Acupuncture, regular massage, and stretching are all common treatments for stiffness and adhesions. After a treatment, it helps to soak in alternating hot and cold baths for the next week. If your muscles are sore and the weather is damp and cold, be sure to stay warm and dry. Keep moving to prevent blood stagnation and stiffness.

Summary

In this chapter, we covered more injuries athletes can get besides the six most common ones. Some of them are similar to injuries already described, but their slight differences warrant a separate explanation. Some of the most effective points for injuries like neck pain can't actually be cupped because they're on your head, and most people have some hair there. Unless you're willing to shave it all off, acupressure or acupuncture should be performed instead of cupping. Acupressure you can do yourself; acupuncture should always be done by a professional.

There were also some conditions that *should never* receive cupping, like a stress fracture. If you aren't sure if your health problem can be cupped, be sure to check before attempting treatment. As with the other sports injuries, try to follow the other recommended treatment options like diet changes and herbal formulations to support cupping's effectiveness.

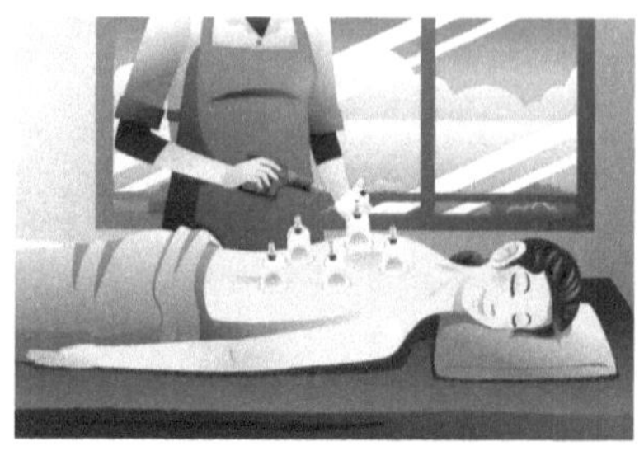

Chapter 7

Athlete-Related Health Conditions

The last chapter covered injuries that athletes often face, but there are other health problems that can arise from being active. Stress from competitions and pain can lead to anxiety, insomnia, and depression. Female athletes deal with irregular periods or amenorrhea, which is when menstruation stops altogether. Then there's nausea, exercise-induced asthma, and more. In this chapter, we'll cover these conditions and provide guides on cupping and other treatment options.

Anxiety

Athletes are frequently under a lot of stress. Workout goals and competitions can take a toll, and that stress literally poisons the body and weakens the spirit. Stress can manifest as nervousness, headaches, insomnia, nausea, and more. These resulting health problems derail an athlete's schedule and makes their life unpleasant. It can threaten their motivation and make them want to quit.

What points should you target?

Pressure points that can relieve anxiety are all over the body. Some of the most effective ones, however, are on the head. UB-10, also known as The Heavenly Pillar, is just below the base of your skull.

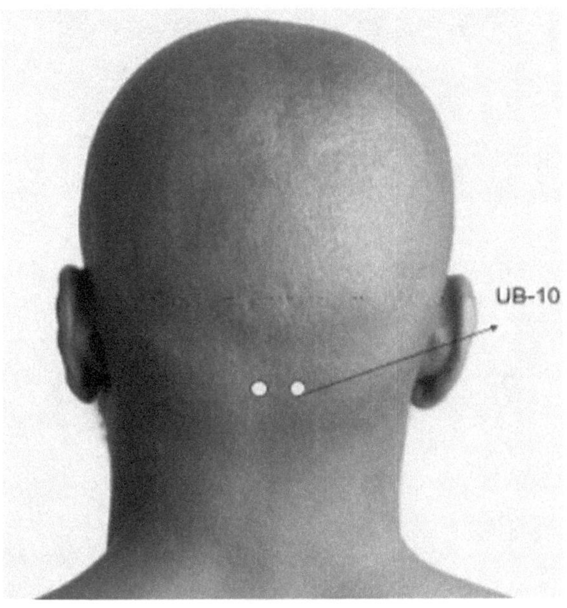

GB-13 may have too much hair to be cupped, so you can apply acupressure instead. Known as GV-24.5, the pressure point right between your eyebrows is very effective at relieving anxiety, headaches, and insomnia. Like all cupping performed on the face, it will be very quick and light, so you don't end up with marks.

Other good points to cup include TB-15, a Triple Burner point, PC-3 and PC-6, HE-7, and CV-17, a point also known as the Sea of Tranquility. It's found in the middle of your breastbone.

Stationary cup on these points for 5-10 minutes and breathe deeply. Use small cups for the points on the head/face and wrist area.

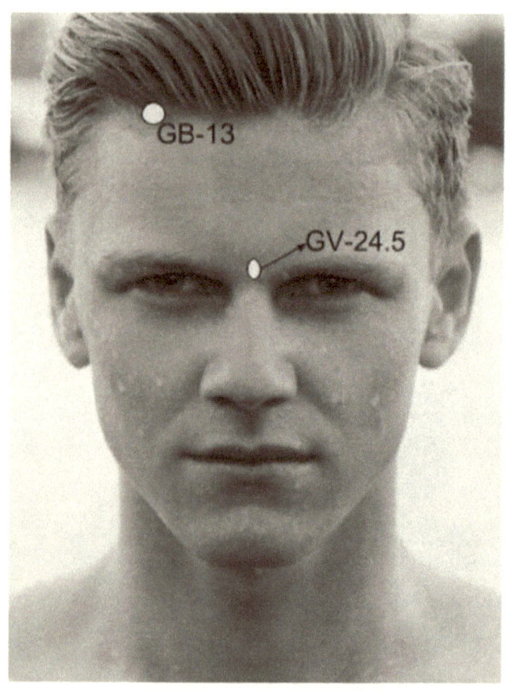

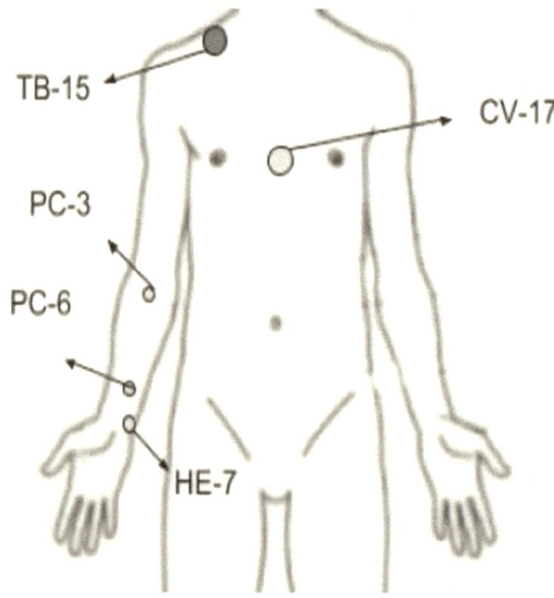

Other treatments for anxiety

Athletes with anxiety often find activities like meditation very relaxing and will practice it regularly as part of their training. Many also find it helpful to talk through their stress with trained professionals and a community they trust and love. For food, seaweed, blueberries, whole grains, and almonds may have anti-anxiety elements. Avoid coffee, soda, and black tea as the high caffeine content increases your heart rate. For herbs, formulations designed to reduce anxiety include ginger, licorice, and white peony root. For short-term help with anxiety, some formulations have calcium and powdered oyster shells. Because these contain heavy metals, they damage the body long-term, so athletes won't use them for very long.

Depression

Frequently paired with anxiety, depression can occur in athletes when they're discouraged about their training, or it can be triggered by something else and affect their training. Depression is so common, there are lots of athletes who have it and it is just a part of their lives. Medications frequently come with lots of side effects, and cupping can help alleviate those symptoms as well as the feelings of hopelessness, fatigue, and sadness that depression triggers.

What points should you target?

The points for depression and anxiety are the same, so just take a look in the section above. In addition to stationary cupping (and flash cupping on the face), therapists might incorporate massage cupping on and around UB-38 in their treatment of depression. This is right over the heart, which is associated with joy. Cupping can also be performed on KI-27, since the kidney meridian is associated with fear. Treating these points can flush those negative emotions from the body.

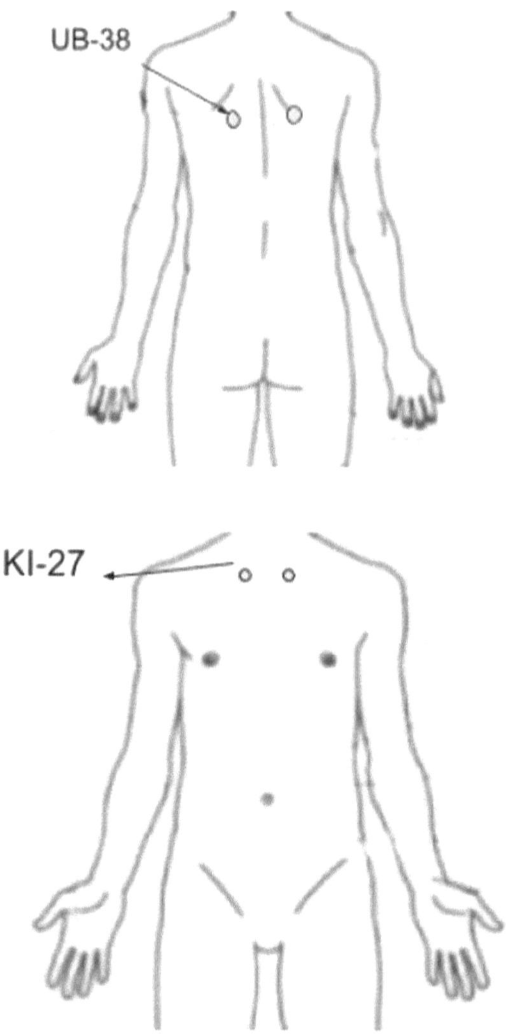

Other treatments for depression

Acupuncture is often performed to treat depression, since there are other points right on the head that you can't cup.

Therapists will also recommend positive, relaxing activities that bring joy. Meditation and exercise are all known to promote the feeling of wellness. For nutrition, foods containing omega-3 fatty acids and complex carbs can help. There has also been a link between vitamin B12 deficiencies and depression, so eat more eggs, poultry, yogurt, and cottage cheese. You can also find almond milk fortified with B12. If you're interested in herbal medicine, formulations will seek to treat the heart and liver. Ingredients like white peony root, ginger, licorice, and even powdered fossils and oyster shells are common. Since fossils and oyster shells contain calcium and heavy metals, they are only intended for short-term use.

Asthma

Even if you don't normally have breathing problems or asthma, exercise can often trigger it. This is known as exercise-induced asthma or exercise-induced bronchoconstriction. Working out causes your airways to narrow, leading to trouble breathing. This is different than regular asthma, which has other factors that affect breathing. Athletes who spend long periods of time breathing deeply, like soccer players, swimmers, and long-distance runners, are the most vulnerable.

Exercise-induced asthma can also be caused by cold and/or dry air, air pollution, a high pollen count, chlorine, chemicals, or lung disease. If you experience coughing, shortness of breath, wheezing, chest tightness, and fatigue, you probably have exercise-induced asthma. It can lead to decreased performance.

What points should you target?

Though exercise-induced asthma is a bit different than regular asthma, you can cup the same pressure points since the symptoms are the same. KI-27 is found under the collarbone and cupping it can relieve chest pain, shortness of breath, and coughing. It also treats anxiety, which often accompanies the feeling that you can't breathe. LU-1 treats asthma, wheezing, and coughing. ST-13, also known as the Qi Door, can be found right under the collar bone between the breastbone and shoulder. It's very close to KI-27. Cupping this point relieves chest heaviness, coughing, and diaphragm spasms. The last point, LU-6, will be cupped especially if your exercise-induced asthma is related to a lung disease. Cupping it relieves coughing.

Your therapist might also apply massage cupping around the lung area of your chest after applying oil.

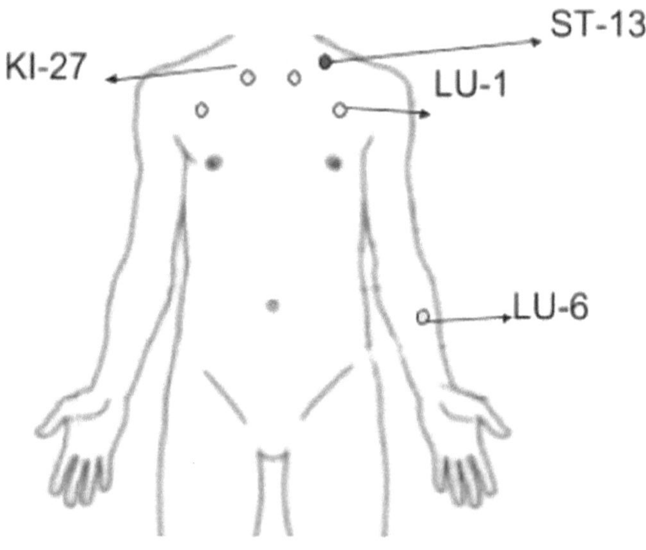

Other treatments for asthma

Acupuncture and acupressure will most likely be applied in addition to cupping. Aromatherapy can also be very helpful, especially with essentials oils like lavender, peppermint, and eucalyptus. For herbal treatments, your therapist will work to figure out what is contributing your asthma. Is it cold, dry air? Is it excessive phlegm? Your lungs and kidney might be weakened, so then herb formulations that increase qi in those organs will be recommended. For your diet, avoid dairy products as they increase phlegm production. Do eat more vitamin B6, which you can find in nuts, seafood, eggs, and legumes. Depending on how severe your asthma is, you might need to carry an inhaler for emergencies.

Insomnia

Sleep is essential to good health. Insomnia is when you have trouble falling asleep, staying asleep, and don't get enough quality REM sleep to actually refresh your body. This sleeping disorder can be caused by a variety of issues, including stress, your schedule, and poor sleep habits. Athletes may experience insomnia because of travel, stress about a competition, or stress about life in general. Athletes are regular people with regular problems, and that can affect sleep. The consequences include fatigue during workouts, decreased performance, anxiety, depression, and a lowered immune system.

Symptoms of insomnia include lying awake at night, waking up during the night, waking up too early, not feeling refreshed when you wake up, fatigue during the day, and trouble concentrating.

What points should you target?

In Traditional Chinese Medicine, many of the pressure points that treat insomnia also treat anxiety, since the goal is to calm the body. PC-6, H7, UB-10, GV-24.5, and CV-17 can be cupped to relieve insomnia and anxiety. Take a look at the anxiety section to see the location of these points. Other points include UB-38, which you can find on the back over the heart. Therapists might apply massage cupping over this point.

GV-16 is at the back of the head, so you'll probably just apply acupressure there and not cupping. GB-20 is very close to UB-10 and can also receive acupressure. The last two points are actually found on the foot. KI-6 and UB-62 can receive stationary cupping with small silicone cups.

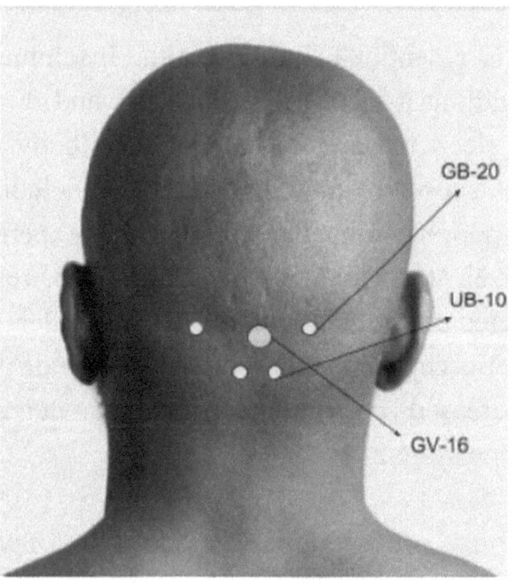

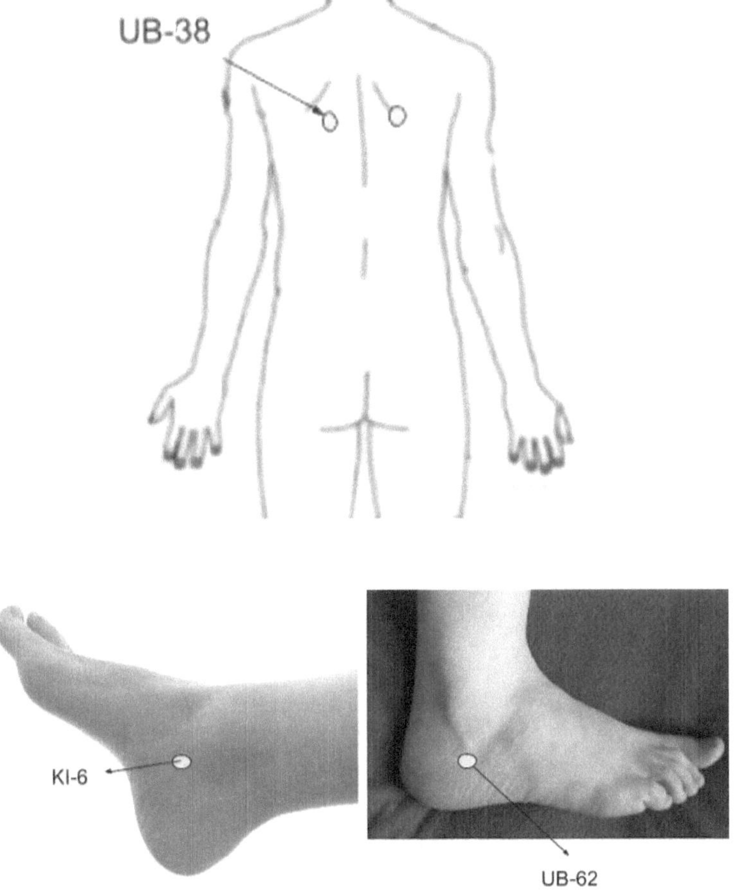

Other treatments for insomnia

Employing good bedtime routines is essential for combating insomnia. Starting to wind down an hour before actually getting into bed helps the mind and body become calm. Turn off electronics and engage in a relaxing ritual, like a warm shower or reading. To encourage good blood circulation (which in turn encourages sleep), soak your feet in hot water until your forehead just breaks a sweat. Be sure the bedroom is completely dark, so your body can produce melatonin.

For food, it's best to avoid eating right before bedtime. About an hour beforehand during your wind-down time, however, certain foods can help your body produce melatonin. Cherries and tart cherry juice are especially good. In Traditional Chinese Medicine, insomnia is often linked to a yin deficiency, so herbs will target the liver, spleen, and heart. Herbal formulations will include licorice root, angelica, and red dates. Herbal teas can also help calm the spirit, though you should avoid black tea and anything with caffeine.

Can you exercise before bed? For some people, it does help, while for others, it gets them too stimulated. An increased heart rate and body temperature can make sleep difficult. You also shouldn't engage in intense cardio workouts, no matter how exercise in general affects your sleep. If you do work out at night, try to time it so it's about 2 hours before bedtime.

Sports-induced anemia

Anemia in athletes is often misdiagnosed as "true anemia," but there is actually a difference. Sports-induced anemia occurs when the athlete's iron store is too low to support their performance. Athletic anemia can develop when red blood cells are destroyed at a fast rate, hemoglobin synthesis is too low, or iron stores aren't high enough or aren't absorbed well enough. It most commonly occurs when, at the beginning of their workout, athletes experience a decreased concentration of hemoglobin, which is the part of red blood cells rich in iron. As a result of sports-induced anemia, athletes lose a lot of iron. Some studies show that this type of anemia may have benefits, but if a person's iron is too low, they actually develop true anemia. When athletes increase their exercise intensity, they can develop sports anemia.

If an athlete isn't eating enough iron, VItamin B12, folic acid, and Vitamin C, they are vulnerable to sports anemia. Certain athletes are more susceptible than others. Women are more likely to get it because of blood loss during their periods. Vegetarian athletes limit their iron intake by eating meat, and vegetarian sources aren't as well-absorbed by the body. Endurance athletes are also at risk because they lose a lot of iron from sweating and from intestinal bleeding.

Symptoms of athletic anemia are the same as true anemia, which is why it's misdiagnosed so often. Athletes will experience fatigue, weakness, shortness of breath, leg cramps, dizziness, or even palpitations.

What points should you target?

Cupping for sports-induced anemia uses the same points as true anemia, since the problem is still found in the blood. Many of the points will target the kidneys, because they are the organs that facilitate red blood cells, which need iron. UB-23 tonifies yang and nourishes yin. GV-4, known as the Ming Men point, is right between the kidneys on the back. CV-4 and ST-36 improve the body's qi.

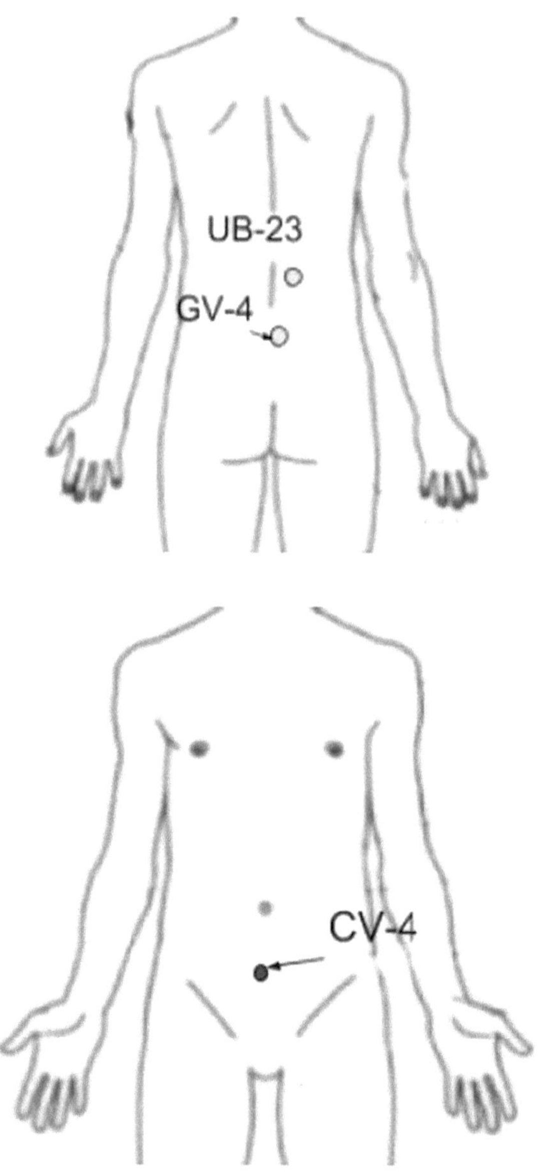
UB-23
GV-4
CV-4

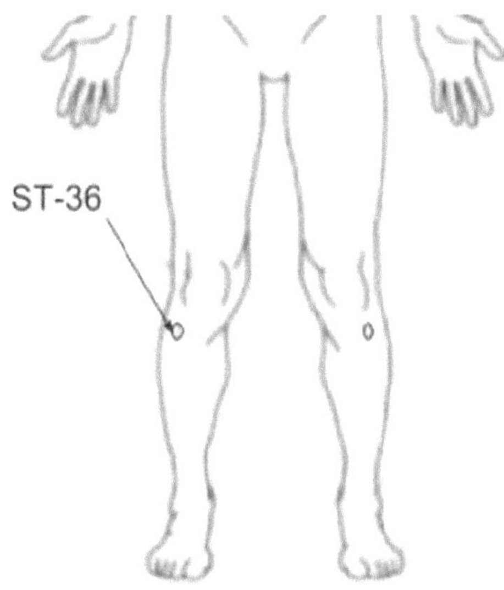

Other treatments for sports-induced anemia

The best treatment for athletic anemia is to increase your iron intake. A therapist might recommend more lean cuts of red meat and dark poultry, as well as enriched and fortified breads and cereals. Vitamin C helps the body absorb iron, while you should avoid foods that inhibit absorption, like coffee and tea. Depending on the severity of your anemia, you might need a supplement. Your training workout might also need an adjustment, with intense workouts spaced out to give the body time to replenish.

In Traditional Chinese Medicine, anemia is believed to be caused by a yin deficiency, so herbs and other treatments will work to address that issue. Dang Shen and Bu Zhong Yi Wan can be helpful, as these herbs boost hemoglobin production. Traditional Chinese Medicine practitioners might also recommend acupuncture.

Nausea

There are a few things that can cause nausea in athletes, though most of the time it's dehydration. This is easily fixed by drinking more water. However, there are other causes like low blood sugar, eating too much before working out, anxiety, and even overhydration. Intense workouts are also known to cause nausea even if the athlete is hydrated, since a rapid heart rate causes blood flow to leave the stomach. Pushing yourself too far or ending an exercise session without a proper cool down (leading to overheating) can also cause that sick feeling.

What points should you target?

If you experience nausea during or after workouts, there are certain points you can cup to reduce the unpleasant feeling. The most convenient points are on your arms, hands, legs, and feet. LI-4 is considered the most effective point and can be found between your thumb and index finger. You'll use a very small cup for just 3-4 minutes. The other point is on your wrist and is known as PC-6, or the Inner Gate. PC-3 is inside the elbow.

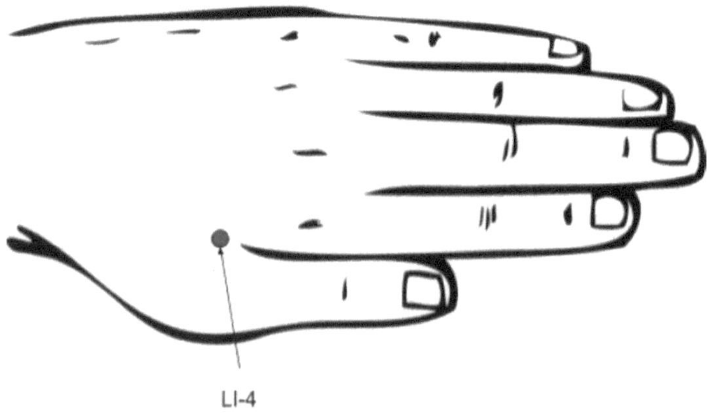

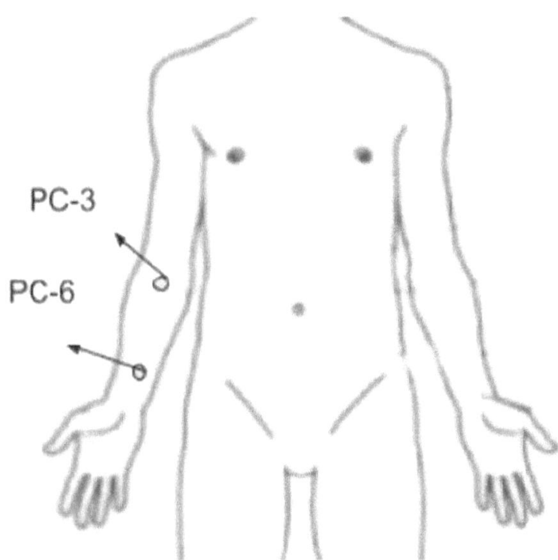

ST-36 is underneath your knee on the outside of the leg by the shinbone. ST-44 is between your second and third toe. If cupping that point is awkward, just apply firm acupressure for a few minutes. In the image, the woman is a little short of the point, you should cup right on the dot.

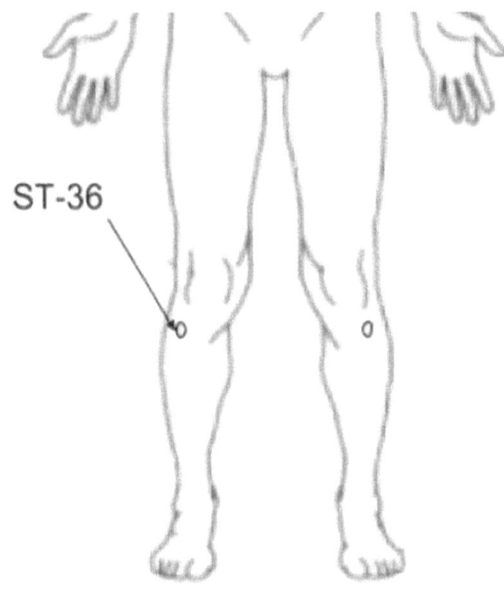

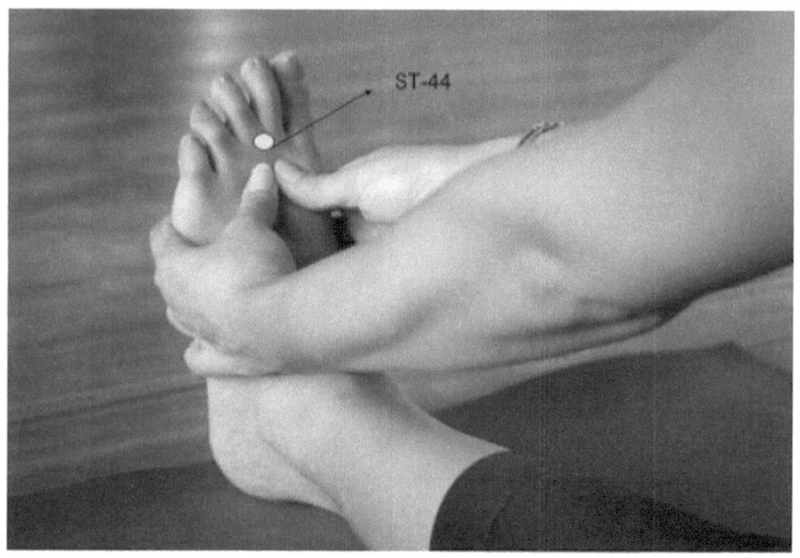

Other treatments for nausea

The best treatment for nausea depends on the cause. If you have signs of dehydration like dry mouth, a headache, dry skin, and dizziness, you should drink water right away. If it's low blood sugar, eat something with salt like pretzels. Chocolate milk with a little salt is a popular recovery drink. Tea made from certain herbs are known to reduce nausea, such as ginger and chamomile. Peppermint is also effective. Your therapist might also recommend herbal formulations with ingredients like ginger, cardamom, and licorice root.

Athlete's foot

Athlete's foot is common among athletes because they spend time in locker rooms and communal showers. This is the perfect environment for the fungus that causes athlete's foot (dermatophyte), because it grows in warm, moist environments. It likes to live between a person's toes and eats dead skin.

What points should you target?

With cupping, you will not actually apply cups to the affected area. Instead, a therapist will identify *why* you got the fungus and what weakness in your body made you vulnerable to the infection. According to Traditional Chinese Medicine, athlete's foot is caused by either a damp-wind invasion or a wind-heat invasion. An imbalance in the body let this external invasion in. The imbalance is usually excess dampness, damp-heat in your body, weak blood circulation, and/or weak qi. The points you'll target relate specifically to the organs that will be comprised. For driving out liver and gallbladder damp-heat, you can cup on ST-40, UB-20, TB-6, and CV-12.

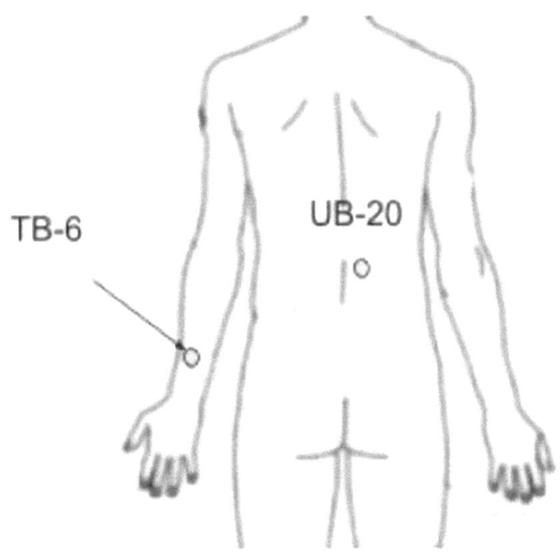

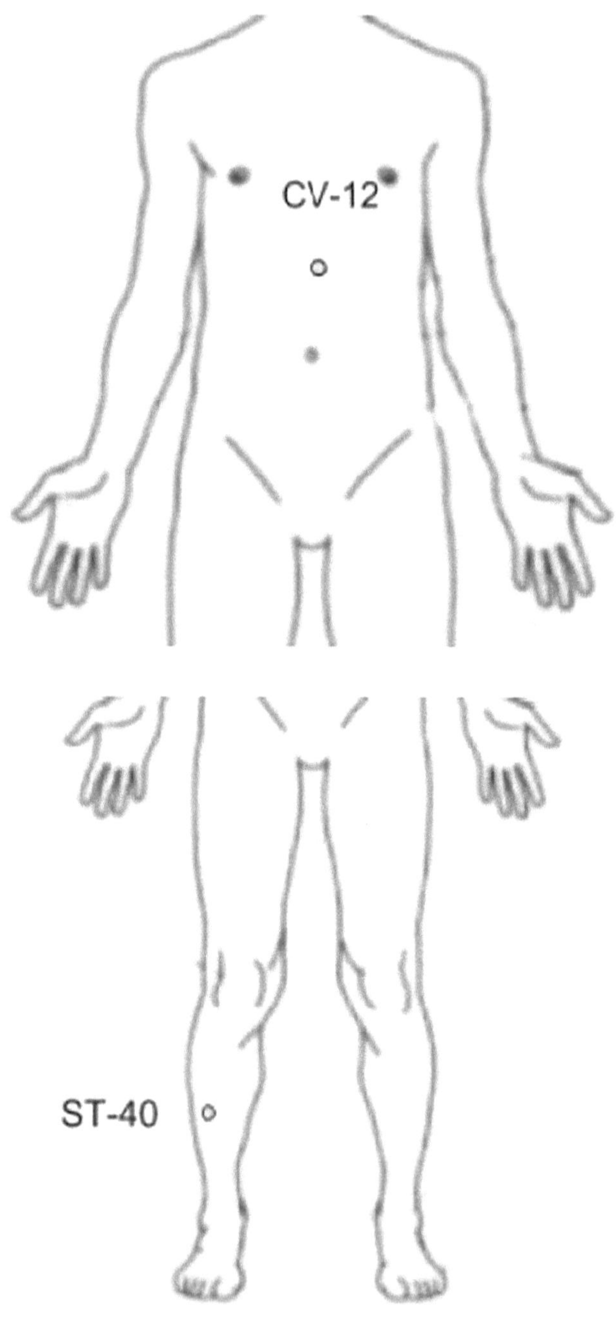

CV-12
ST-40

To drive out liver wind, cup LV-3 and GB-20. They help improve qi stagnation and drive out wind from the head. For spleen and stomach damp heat, there are six key points. ST-44 and LI-11 cool heat; LI-11 also relieves dampness and is used for treating other skin conditions. SP-9 relieves dampness and ST-36 and UB-20 strengthens the spleen. CV-12 regulates qi.

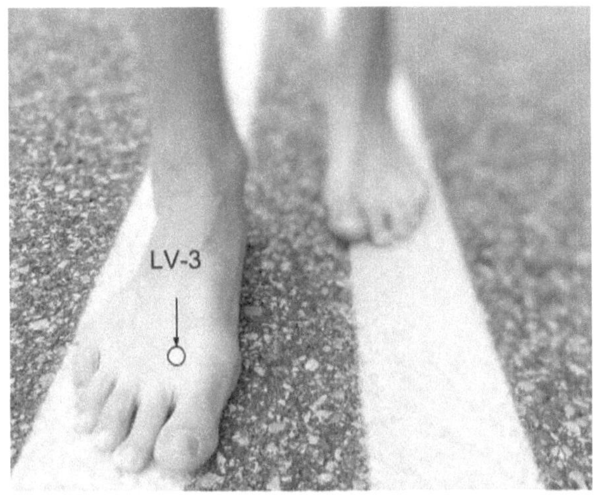

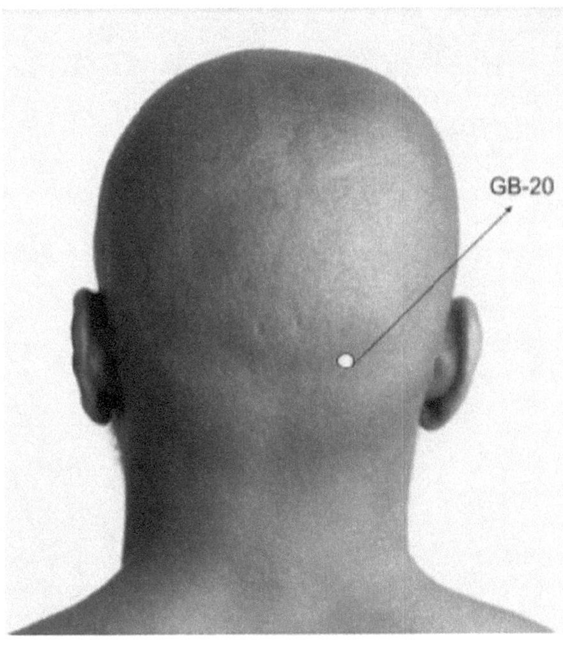

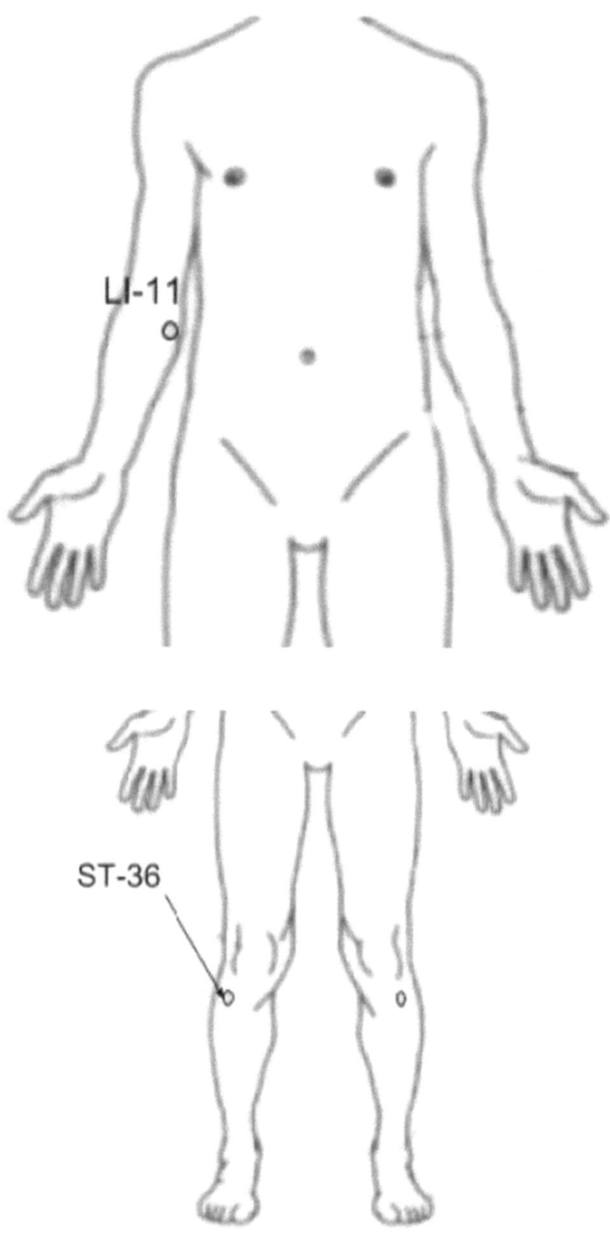

LI-11
ST-36

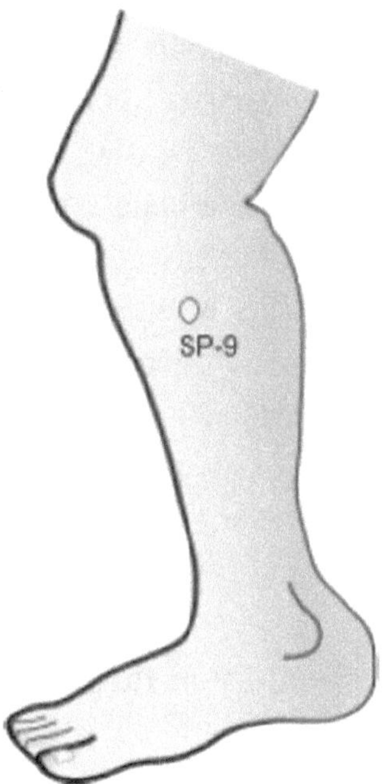

Other treatments for athlete's foot

The most common treatment for athlete's foot is a cream, so therapists might recommend one with natural ingredients that helps to stimulate blood flow, as well. Creams with harsh ingredients like soap, rubbing alcohol, iodine, and hydrogen peroxide can irritate your skin further. Soaking your feet in water and diluted tea tree oil for five minutes twice a day should clear up the fungus in a few weeks, depending on how bad the infection is.

In terms of your diet, you should avoid foods with "dampening" qualities, like fruit juices, tropical fruit, tofu, shellfish, and fatty fish. Avoid wearing thick socks and stay dry as much as possible. Cotton is the best material. If your feet sweat a lot, use a body powder to keep the area dry.

Skin rashes

Because of the close contact with other people, sharing equipment, and environments like locker rooms, athletes frequently come down with skin rashes and infections. Wrestlers often spread ringworm, while athlete's foot (which we discussed above) can occur for just about any athlete. Athletes can also come down with heat rash, which is when sweat glands are blocked and sweat can't evaporate. The skin becomes inflamed and breaks out into a rash. "Jock itch," which is a tinea infection in the groin, occurs when there's a lot of sweating in the area or if you don't change out of wet clothes after swimming. Men are nearly always the ones to get this infection.

What points should you target?

You actually *should not* perform cupping on rashes. Covering the irritation and creating suction further aggravates the area. There are much more effective and safer treatment options.

Other treatments for skin rashes

Acupuncture will be performed instead of cupping, though needles aren't inserted in the affected areas. Instead, the therapist will treat the root of the problem and the relevant organ. For herbs, Three Yellow Powder with its cooling ingredients is the most popular and used for 60% of all skin disorders. Other herbs will be decided based on what the specific diagnosis is. Skin itchiness can be caused by a variety of factors, such as internal infections, overheated blood, accumulated dampness, and wind-heat.

Menstruation disorders

Irregular or missed periods are a common health condition among female athletes who are very active. The official condition is known as hypothalamic amenorrhea, and it means that you've missed your period for more than 6 months. Doctors aren't quite sure why this develops; the understanding used to be it was because athletes are too lean, but that may not be accurate.

Instead, irregular and missed periods may be because of body weight and not the amount of body fat. Women who fall below 85-90% of the ideal body weight for their height - regardless of fat levels - are much more likely to get amenorrhea. Poor nutrition also plays a role. Not having a period means your production of estrogen goes down, leading to bone thinness. For athletes, this is especially concerning because they will be more susceptible to injuries.

An athlete's period may not stop completely, but can become irregular. A regular period occurs every 28-30 days and lasts between 3 days and one week. Irregular periods can cause bloating and cramping at random times during the month, and the days between cycles are never the same. In addition to the lack of a period, symptoms of hypothalamic amenorrhea include a low libido, insomnia, low energy, and increased hunger.

What points should you target?

The issues causing irregular and missed periods are the same, so cupping can be performed on the same points for both disorders. The cupping treatment is usually applied 3-5 days before bleeding actually begins, which can be tricky when you don't know when your period will be. Cupping will also be performed 2 days after bleeding stops. For patients not having periods at all, it can be performed anytime.

Points are spread around the body, so you'll be cupping on the belly, hands, and legs.
CV-3 and CV-6 can be lightly cupped or massaged. These points also help relieve menstrual cramps and constipation. SP-6, SP-10, LI-3, and LI-4 can be stationary cupped for 5-10 minutes. LI-3 is between the thumb and first finger when your hand is relaxed, before the webbing. Moxibustion often follows to further warm the area.

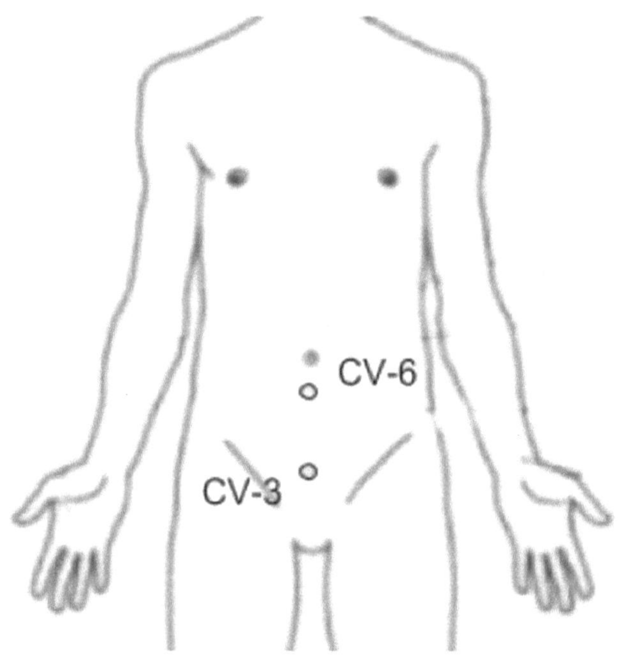

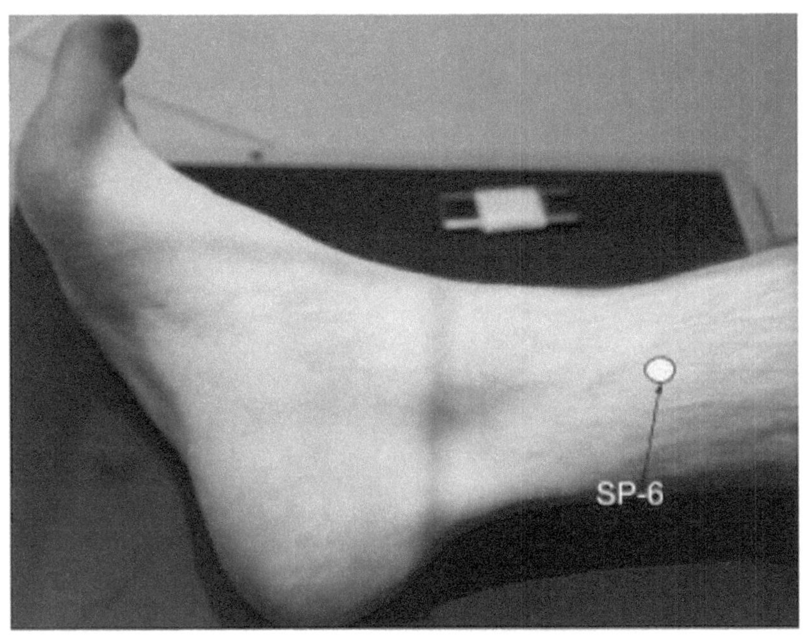
SP-6

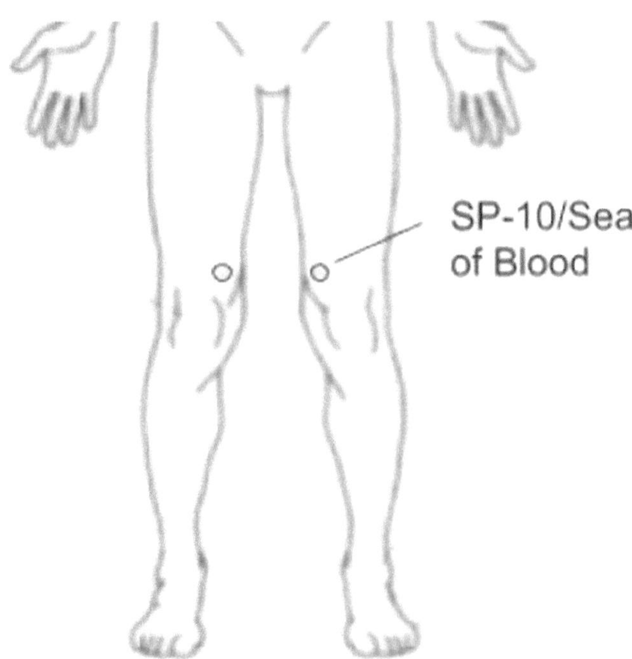
SP-10/Sea
of Blood

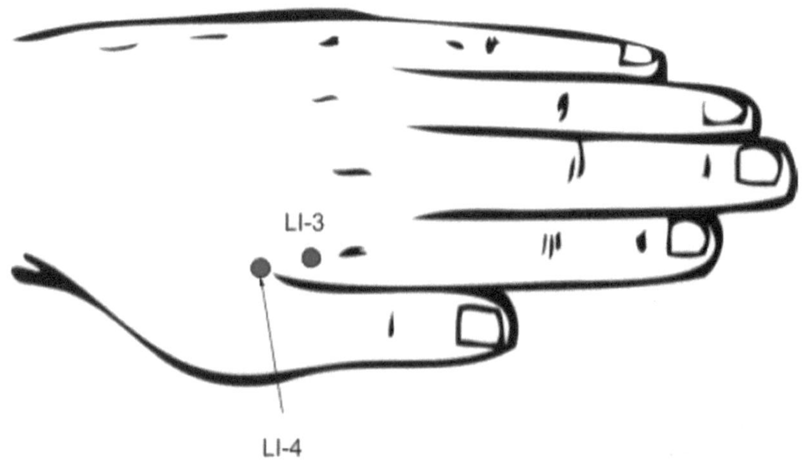

Other treatments for menstrual disorders

Since there are so many possible causes for irregular or missed periods, a therapist will customize treatment based on the individual. For athletes, it's not as if they can necessarily just "put on more fat" to stop the problem. If the problem lies within the kidney and liver, you might experience fatigue, soreness and weakness in your legs and groin, lower back pain, dizziness, anxiety, hot flashes, and frequent urination. A problem with the qi and blood leads to dizziness, palpitations, headaches, loose bowel movements, weakness, insomnia, and breathlessness.

Therapists also believe qi stagnation, blood stasis, and phlegm dampness can cause irregular and eventually missed periods. Qi stagnation symptoms include depression, anxiety, headaches, breast tenderness, lack of appetite, and alternating bouts of constipation and diarrhea. Blood stasis, in addition to irregular and missed periods, manifests as headaches, depression, breast tenderness, and otherwise more painful symptoms than qi stagnation. Phlegm dampness is more common for people who are overweight and who eat cold, raw, and greasy food, so it doesn't happen often in athletes. Symptoms include nausea, headaches, phlegm caught in the throat, bloating, fatigue, and weakness.

Acupuncture is often performed, which activates qi and removes toxins and blocks from the body's meridians. The spleen and conception vessel are especially important. A therapist might also recommend eating more freshwater shrimp, black beans, red dates, and other foods high in iron. Raw, cold, and spicy food should be avoided, as should alcohol and caffeine.

Depending on what the specific root problem is, the therapist will recommend herbal formulations with ingredients like angelica, Chinese yam, white peony, ginseng, and astragalus.

Liver deficiency due to overtraining

When athletes overtrain with little recovery time or rest, their muscles weaken, leading to tendon problems. In turn, this tendon weakness causes imbalances in the liver blood. There might already be problems there, but overtraining aggravates it. Liver blood represents the yin part of the liver, so overtraining directly leads to yin deficiency. If not treated, liver blood imbalances can lead to Liver Wind, which is an internal Wind/Evil. Symptoms include dizziness, pulsing headaches, neck stiffness, tremors, limb numbness, and fainting spells.

What points should you target?

To tonify your liver blood, cup on ST-36, SP-6, LI-4, LV-3, and LV-8. If your therapist determines the root of the problem is yin deficiency in your liver, they'll pay special attention to LV-8.

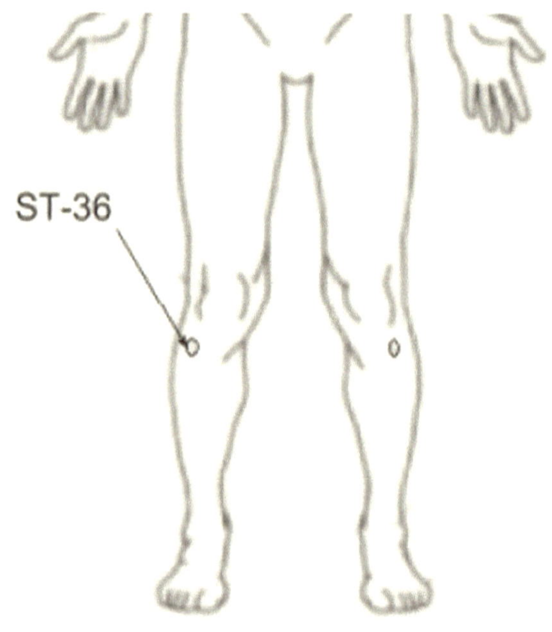

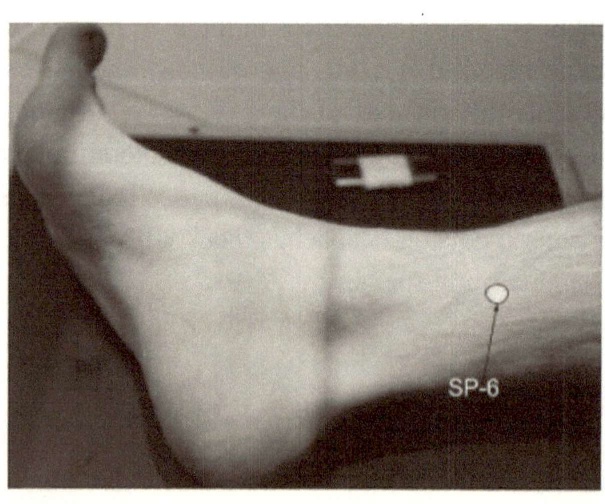

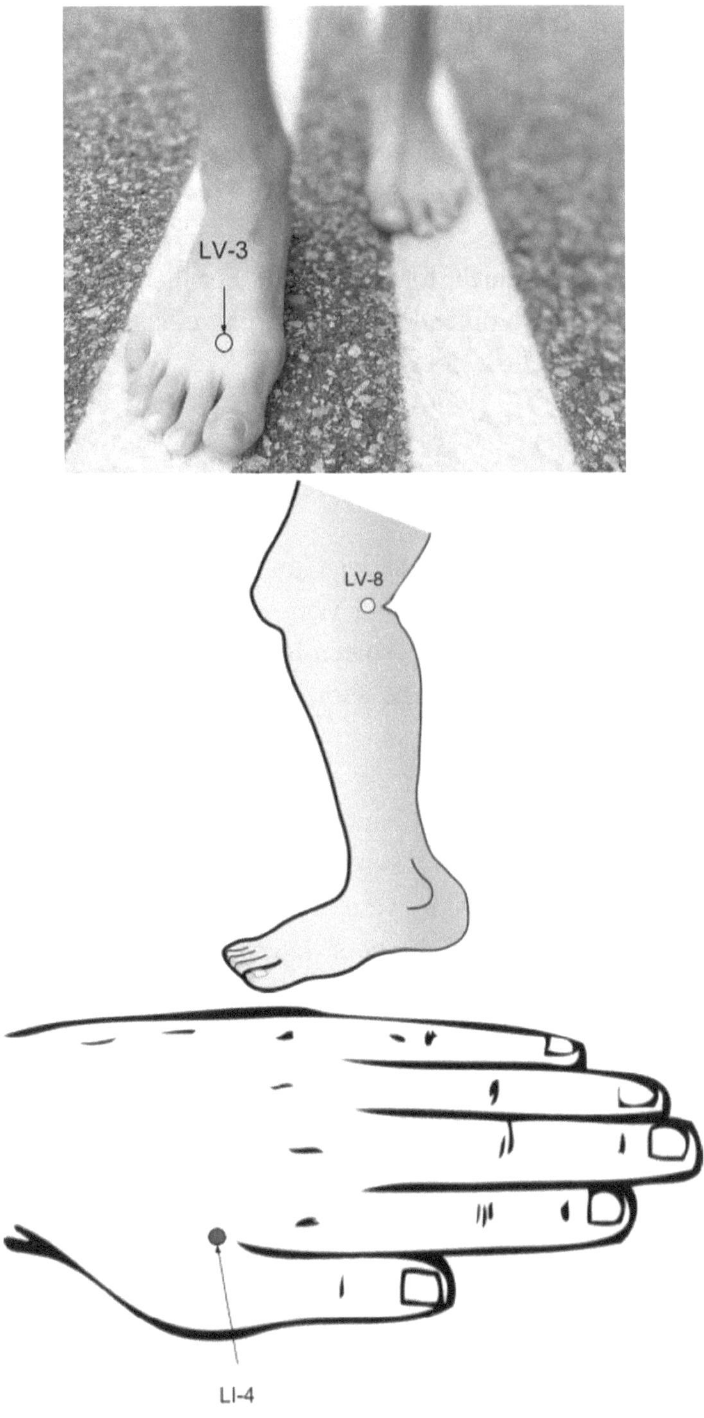
LV-3
LV-8
LI-4

Other treatments for liver deficiency

A change in diet can have a significant impact on the problem. Plants like mung beans and sprouts, millet, and dark leafy greens are all recommended. Fruits like blueberries, blackberries, and raspberries are also helpful. Drinkable aloe vera is considered one of the best tonics for liver yin. For herbal formulations, therapists will recommend ones with ingredients like angelica, peony root, and yellow dock root.

Kidney deficiency due to overtraining

Overtraining can also lead to kidney deficiency. This is concerning because the yin and yang energies of *the whole body* come from the kidneys. The spleen is especially affected, because the spleen and kidneys are closely related and have similar functions.

When your kidneys become deficient, both yin and yang deplete with one another. Symptoms of yin deficiency include dizziness, problems with your hearing, constipation, sudden sweating, and weakness in your knees and lower back. Yang deficiency manifests as soreness and a cold feeling in your knees and lower back, trouble peeing, weakness, and cold limbs.

What points should you target?

There are specific points for kidney qi, ying, and yang deficiency, but because these are all so closely-related, a therapist might perform cupping on all of them. Tonifying one tonifies the other. For yin, cup ST-36 and KI-9. For yang, ST-36, KI-2, and KI-7. For overall qi, point KI-3 can be added.

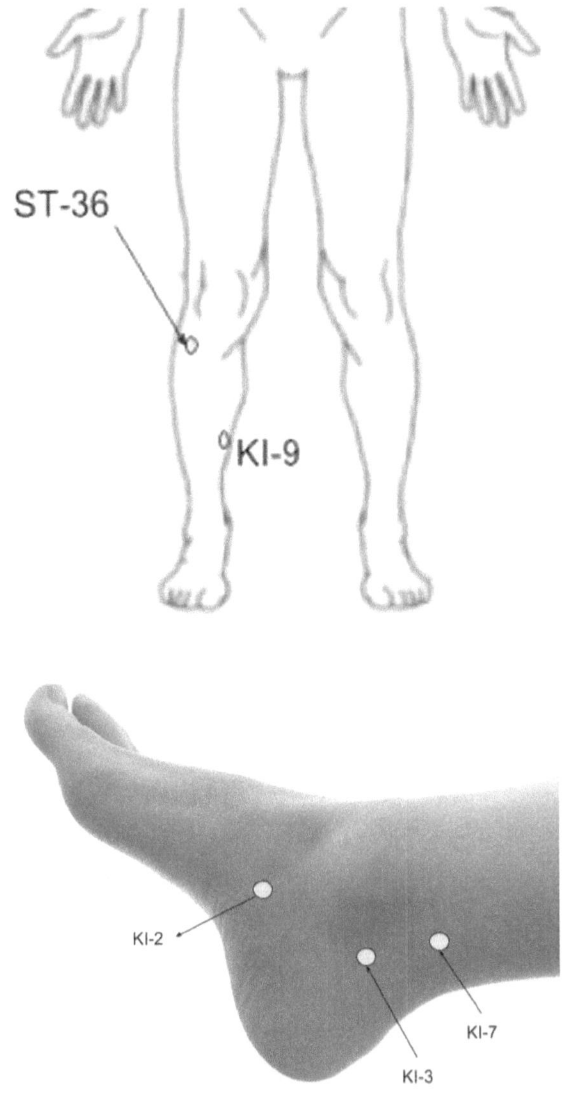

Other treatments for kidney deficiency

Acupuncture is a common treatment either alongside cupping or as a replacement. Diet and herbal formulations can help deal with the problem, too. Your therapist might recommend more vegetables, lean proteins, carrots, walnuts, salmon, dates, and garlic. Herb formulations that tonify your kidney qi will include reishi mushrooms, fenugreek, cinnamon bark, jiaogulan, and cornus.

Spleen deficiency due to overtraining

A deficiency of spleen qi is very common for athletes. The spleen (and stomach) is the seat of the body's qi and blood. If these aren't working properly, it affects your whole body's qi. While people in general often have reduced qi in their spleens, athletes are especially vulnerable because of their busy and physically-exhausting lifestyles. Athletes dealing with the pressure of school are the most susceptible since they often are not eating properly. They will experience digestive issues, muscle weakness, fatigue, and a lack of concentration.

What points should you target?

Pressure points include SP-3 and SP-6, which both tonify the qi. UB-20 and UB-21 are also effective, as is ST-36. Moxibustion can be performed after cupping.

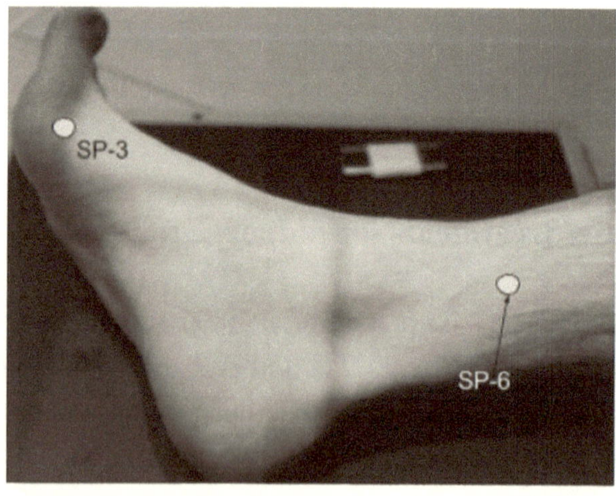

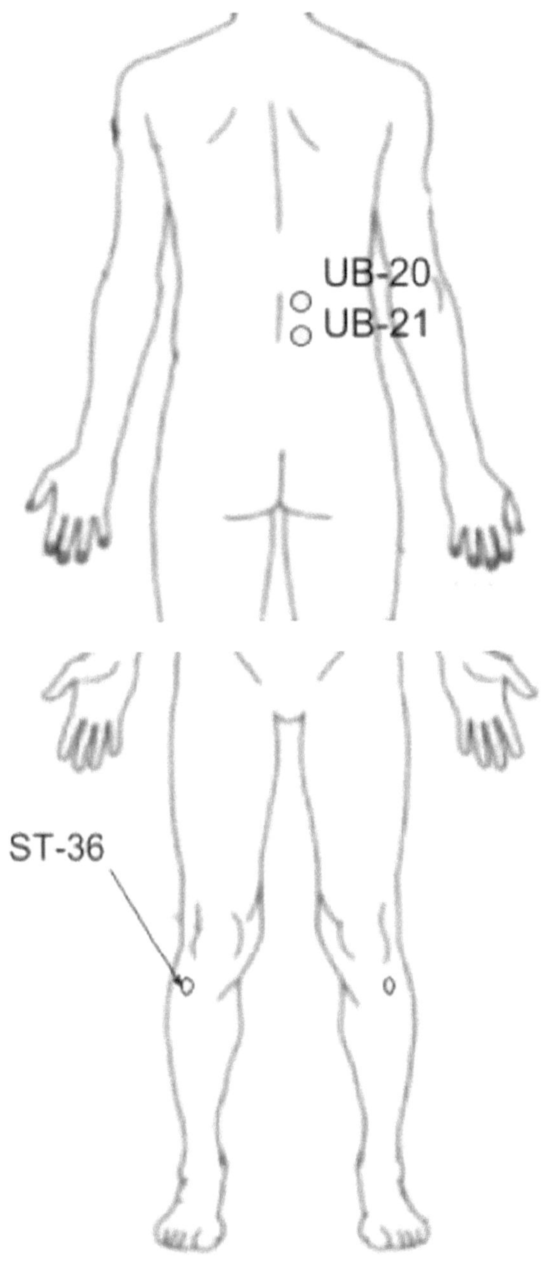
UB-20
UB-21
ST-36

Other treatments for spleen deficiency

Like most problems, acupuncture can be added to a cupping treatment or used in its place. Since spleen deficiency eventually leads to dampness, recommended foods and herbs will deal with that. Rosemary, garlic, dried ginger, lamb, shrimp, walnuts, and raspberries are all good choices. Jasmine and peppermint tea can also increase qi. Any sweet and pungent flavors are good, since they encourage qi circulation through the body. Avoid excess sugar and salt, as well as dairy products, gluten, citrus fruits, tofu, pork, and bananas. Herbal formulations will include ingredients like astragalus and ginseng.

Underperformance syndrome

The name is vague because there doesn't appear to be any specific medical reason to why it happens. An athlete suddenly becomes tired all of the time, has a weakened immune system, changes in their resting heart rate, and trouble sleeping. Odds are, they are working themselves too hard. However, if an athlete experiences fatigue and decreased performance after 2 weeks of rest, a therapist will look at the patient's tongue for clues. According to Traditional Chinese Medicine, here's what the different options mean:

Pale-colored tongue
Diagnosis: Low qi

If the tongue is also dry and thin, it's a blood deficiency.
If it's wet, it's qi deficiency.
If it's swollen, it's also qi deficiency.
If the tongue is wet *and* swollen, it's a yang deficiency.

Pink-colored tongue
Diagnosis: Healthy or a mild disorder

Red-colored tongue
Diagnosis: Excessive body heat

If the tongue is also yellow, it means you have excess heat in your body.
If the tongue is red and wet, it's a damp heat.
If the tongue is red and dry, you have some kind of injury.

Dark-red tongue
Diagnosis: Extreme body heat

Purple tongue
Diagnosis: Blood stagnation

Blue-colored tongue
Diagnosis: Severe internal cold

What points should you target?

Your therapist will determine the most effective points based on what they learn about your health. The points will correspond to the most relevant organs, for example, for a purple tongue and blood stagnation, the therapist will most likely target the spleen and kidneys for nourishing; the heart for circulation; and the liver for storage.

Other treatments for underperformance syndrome

Since this condition is relatively mysterious, therapists are sometimes torn between how much rest a patient should get.

Generally, however, it's a good idea to gradually increase your workouts by 5-10 minutes each day. Depending on what the therapist discovers about your health based on their assessment, their recommendations will vary.

To tackle the issue of motivation and lack of energy, there are lots of herbs and herb formulations that can help. Cordyceps can build your stamina and endurance by increasing your body's ability to use oxygen. Reishi mushrooms are said to "calm the spirit," specifically the nervous system, so your tolerance to stress increases. It also strengthens the immune system. Siberian ginseng contains strength-building compounds that affect the lungs and spleens in particular, which are essential for pulling energy from the food you eat. Lastly, schisandra fruit, a dried berry, can be made into a tea that regulates your blood pressure, stabilizes blood sugar levels, and improves your resistance to stress.

For your diet, try drinking yerba mate tea, which is an excellent coffee substitute since it contains less harmful caffeine. It provides energy without shocking the system. You can also try shots of wheatgrass and apple cider vinegar. For food, snack on raw almonds, seeds, bananas, and broccoli for more magnesium.

Summary

The conditions in this chapter were ones that don't necessarily stem from athletic activity, but they can certainly affect an athlete's life. Whether it's anxiety before a competition, a rash from sweating, or trouble sleeping, cupping can provide relief. Certain conditions - mainly rashes and athlete's foot - should only be cupped on distal points since the therapy can actually irritate the condition further. Other treatments like a change in diet and herbs will help healing and strength-building.

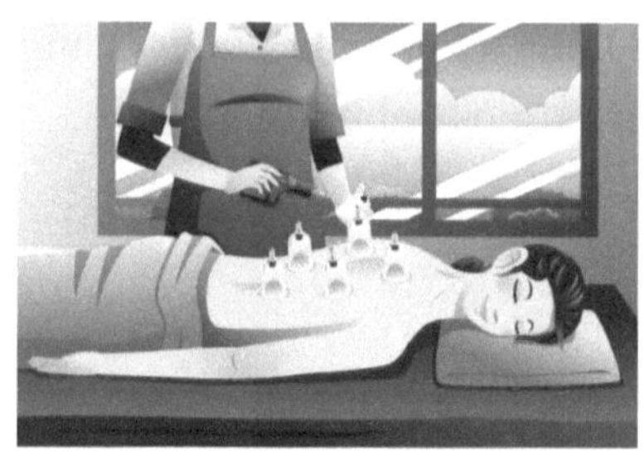

C h a p t e r   8

What to Remember

This book had a lot of information on cupping and what it can do for a wide variety of health conditions that athletes face. What are the most important takeaways you should remember before pursuing this type of therapy?

Cupping isn't a one-stop shop for health

Cupping has been used for centuries for health problems like neck pain, pulled and strained muscles, anxiety, and more, but it's rarely performed by itself. Other treatments like acupuncture, moxibustion, and herbal medicine are just as important, and together, they enhance one another's benefits. You also need to take care of your body through diet and exercise adjustments if necessary; if you don't, cupping probably won't be very effective. Traditional Chinese Medicine is all about caring for the whole body from the inside out, and not just the symptoms.

Cupping isn't widely-accepted by the scientific or general medical community

Many doctors in the West don't believe cupping is a legitimate medical treatment. Some are even opposed to it, believing it deceives patients and may lead to them refusing other care. There aren't studies that show cupping is dangerous, however, the issue is that cupping just hasn't been studied very much. It's very challenging to test cupping because the standard process is to use a control group and placebo, and you can't "fake" cupping. Data will always be filtered through some kind of bias. In countries where cupping is practiced in hospitals, like China, it does have support.

Cupping comes with risks

Cupping is generally safe, but there are risks. This is especially true if you attempt cupping without a professional, and most will recommend that you always seek out treatment from a practitioner. Traditional dry cupping with flame is especially dangerous, and you should *not* try it at home. Cupping with pumps or with bulbed cups is much safer. As a note, if you are cupping for a serious health condition, it is best to seek out a trained professional. If the problem is more superficial or you are already seeking treatment from professionals in some form, cupping is safe and you will probably see positive results.

If cupping at home, be extra careful about meeting hygiene standards and monitoring pain

Speaking of cupping at home, you want to pay special attention to your hygiene standards. Always wash your hands and equipment before, and make sure to sterilize your cups before and after each use.

During a cupping session, you should also monitor the level of discomfort. Pain is never good. Cupping can feel uncomfortable, but it should never be painful. You should stop right away. When starting out, try light cupping first to see how it feels. If you're massage cupping, don't forget to apply oil and use flexible cups.

Know when (and where) you shouldn't cup

Cupping isn't always the appropriate treatment for a health condition. In this book, I described a few issues and ended up telling you that cupping shouldn't be performed. These include rashes, fungal infections, and areas where the pain will be too strong. You also cannot cup on people with fevers, who are weak, who are hungry, or who have a pacemaker. If you can feel a pulse, an artery, or a bone, you don't want to place a cup there.

Always educate yourself before considering cupping

Before heading into a Traditional Chinese Medicine clinic or buying a cupping set, be sure you've done your research well. Cupping doesn't work for everybody and it may not be the best option for you, so you want to talk to your doctor and a cupping therapist first. What questions should you ask your doctor? Some good ones are:

- Am I getting the standard treatments for my health problem? Is there anything I can change in my diet or exercise that could help?
- Is there any medical reason why I shouldn't try cupping?

For the cupping therapist, you want to be sure they're well-trained and well-versed in the condition you would receive cupping for, so ask them:

- Where did you train?
- How experienced are you with cupping and my health condition?
- Would you recommend cupping for me? Or is there another treatment that would be better?

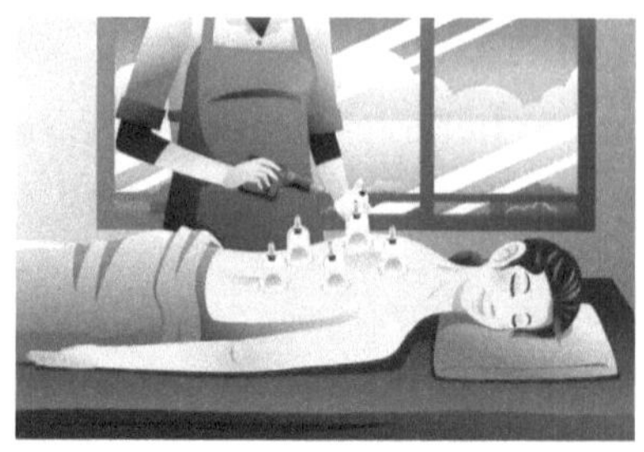

Epilogue

Exercise and athletic activities are very good for the body, but they can take their toll on it too. Improper form, painful falls, and external factors like the environment can cause injuries like strains, sprains, and even internal problems like sports-induced anemia. Traditional Chinese Medicine has dealt with these types of problems for centuries, but for a while, modern medicine ignored the potential benefits. However, athletes have recently embraced cupping as a very effective way to encourage healing and boost good health. It's become common to see those tell-tale circular marks on toned and muscular bodies all over the world.

What is cupping and how is it done? This book answered these questions in chapters on the Traditional Chinese Medicine system, the different types of cupping, and guides on cupping for injuries like ankle sprains, back pain, asthma, and more. The body is made up of meridians or areas controlled and monitored by different organs. By stimulating certain points along these meridians, cupping activates the body's natural healing and detoxifying abilities. This book uses abbreviations for the points that are used universally, so if you aren't sure about where a point is located or you want to learn more, you can look it up.

What kind of cups should you use? Materials include glass, plastic, rubber, and silicone. Plastic, rubber, and silicone are the most popular these days because they're safer, flexible, and easy to clean. Traditional dry cupping uses glass, because suction is created by heat from a fire, and should only be performed by professionals. Other supplies include massage oils, essential oils, and clean towels. If you're cupping at home, you should be extra careful about hygiene.

If you are active at all, you are at risk for injuries. You don't need to be a professional to get hurt, and some injuries can even occur while you're just strolling down the street and slip on a pebble. Cupping can be an effective way to manage pain and speed up recovery if it's done properly, and I am grateful that you read this book as part of your research. If you have more questions about cupping, consult a Traditional Chinese Medicine practitioner in your area, and if you believe you might have one of the health issues described in this book, please make an appointment with your doctor. Stay healthy, stay safe, and stay happy!